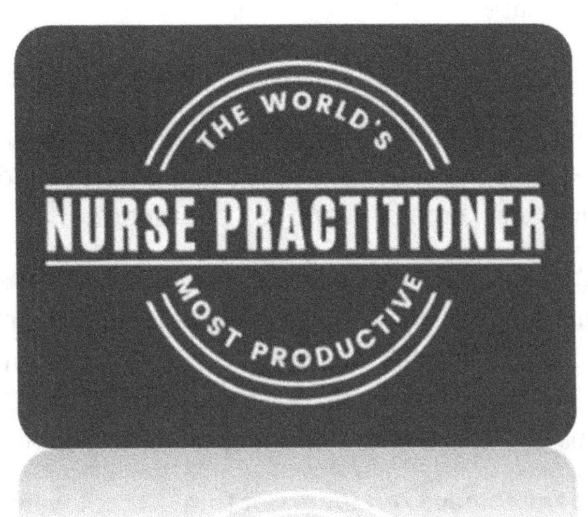

CHEAT SHEETS

Hello and thank you for your purchase!

This notebook consists of the only cheat sheets that are ever really acceptable to use – documentation cheat sheets. I developed these while I was in Nurse Practitioner school and used them in all of my clinical encounters while in school and the first year or so of practice.

These cheat sheets served multiple purposes for me – first, in the simplest sense, they provided a way to quickly and consistently document on the patients that I was seeing in my clinical rotations. I did not have to worry about sharing a computer in the exam room with my preceptor; I could get everything done on my little cheat sheets. I prepped before the visit, circled or crossed out various parts of the subjective and objective sections as I talked with the patient, and added notes in the free text area.

Having these sheets also helped me to have reminders of things that I wanted to be sure to cover depending on the presenting concern for the patient. If I had a patient presenting with dizziness, I might ask questions from the cardiovascular, neurological, and ears/nose/throat sections. Time permitting, before going into the exam room, I would even highlight the sections I wanted to be sure to cover (both the subjective and objective areas). This helped to make me more efficient AND effective in the visit and really boosted my confidence.

Having the information from my documentation cheat sheets made it so much easier to give report to my preceptor. And when it came time to document, I had all of the information that I needed to speed right through charting (and of course, as a student, I had to chart everything twice – once in my preceptor's charting system and again in my school's charting system). At the end of each rotation, I had a nice chunk of notes that I could refer to if necessary – or even look back at and see how far I had come!

In my first year of practice as a Nurse Practitioner, I continued to use these cheat sheets. They were a lifesaver in terms of helping to make sure I always ran on time, asked the right questions, and assessed the right things in the visit. When the time came to chart, I even had my scripts right there in front of me – the content of each body system listed on the cheat sheet is basically what you need in your note ("Patient denies SOB, cough, wheeze"). These were turned into charting shortcuts (called smartphrases in Epic).

Whether you are a student, a new grad, or someone looking to fast-track your charting, I hope these help you feel confident in your clinical encounters and help you run on time and keep your charting robust yet efficient.

Take care,

Jessica

<table>
<tr><td>Patient ID#:</td><td>Date of visit:</td></tr>
<tr><td>Reason for visit:</td><td>Age: Gender:</td></tr>
</table>

BP: HT:
HR: WT:
T: BMI:
O2%:   PAIN:

NOTES . . . .

CONST Δ appetite, energy, weight / fever / chills / sweats / fatigue
HEAD trauma / mass / tenderness / rash / lesions
EYES visionΔ / itch / d/c / tears / dry / cataracts / glaucoma / glasses, contacts
ENT hearing Δ / pain / d/c / vertigo / ? infection // epistaxis / congestion // bleeding, swelling gums / pain / sore throat / voice Δ // neck pain / lumps / swelling / difficulty swallowing

CARDIAC pain / pressure / dizzy / N / orthopnea / edema / palp / weak w exertion / hx murmurs / hx MI / HTN / HF / numb / tingle / cold extrem / slow wound healing

RESP wheeze / SOB / cough / asthma / bronch / COPD
GI abd pain / Δ in bowels / constipation / diarrhea / N V / hepatitis / gallstones / dysphagia / reflux / hemorrhoids / black, bloody stools

GU burn / pain / nocturia / polyuria / hematuria / incontinence / infection / kid. stones
GENITAL DC / sores / pain / masses / last pap _____ / sexually active Y N / dyspareunia / LMP _____ / contraception

MSK redness / swelling / warmth / pain / +/- ROM / arthritis / musc cramps / fracture / sprains / joint replacement / stiffness: AM PM
SKIN rash / pruritis / jaundice / bruising / hx skin ca / mole Δ / Δ in hair, nails / lesions / slow wound healing

BREASTS lump / pain / dc / last mammo _____ / self exams YN
NEURO HA / seizure / vertigo / memory Δ / gait Δ / speech / coord
PSYCH depression / anxiety / Δ in sleep pattern / substance, ETOH abuse / suicidal ideation / homicidal ideation

ENDO polydipsia, polyuria / heat, cold intolerance / Δ hair/nails/energy
HEM/LYMPH anemia / bruising / hx transfusions / blood disorder / lymphadenopathy / axillary, groin tenderness

ALLX/IMMUN season allx / food allx / med allx / immune disorder:

SOCIAL HX # in household _____ / lives with SP/BF/GF/SO / children __ / tobacco Y/N #pk / sexual activity Y/N / etoh, other substances Y/N / occupation:
FAM HX ca / HTN / MI / CAD / stroke / hyperlipidemia / DM2 / Alzheimer's / depression / osteoporosis / other:

GENERAL well appearing / well nourished / a&o x 3 / normal mood / normal affect
NEURO intact / abnormal   **DTR:** 1 2 3 4 5 location:
SKIN + NAILS turgor / rash / bruising / lesions // texture, distribution of hair // nails: abnormal color / nail deformity

HEAD normocephalic / atraumatic / visible mass / palpable mass / depression / scarring
EYES acuity intact / conjunctiva clear / EOM intact / PERRLA / fundi: normal discs and vessels / icterus / exudate / hemorrhage

EARS EACs clear / TM translucent, mobile / landmarks abnormal / hearing diminished
NOSE lesions / mucosal inflammation / septum, turbinates abnormal / sinus tenderness
MOUTH mucous membranes dry / lesions / poor dentition / caries / gingival inflammation
PHARYNX mucosa inflammation / tonsillar hypertrophy / tonsillar exudate
NECK supple / ROM WNL / lesion / bruit / adenopathy / thyroid enlarged, tender / mass
CARDIAC regular rate, rhythm / S1, S2 / murmur / gallop / click / rub / PMI displacement
RESP clear to auscultation in all fields / wheezes (insp) (exp) / rales / crackles
ABDOMEN BSx4 / tender / organomegaly / mass / hernia
RECTAL abnormal tone / hemorrhoids (int/ext) / palpable mass
BACK abnormal curvature / tenderness / CVAT / Δ ROM
EXTREMITIES amputation / deformity / edema / varicosities / + pulses
MSK abnormal gait / asymmetry / crepitation / defect / tenderness / mass / effusion / Δ ROM / instability / atrophy / abnormal strength, tone in head, neck, spine, ribs, pelvis, UE, LE / pathologic reflexes

PSYCH A&O x3 / +recent/remote memory / insight / affect
BREAST nipple abnormality / mass / tenderness / axillary, clavicular adenopathy
GYN/GU lesions / d/c / uterus, adnexa tenderness / CMT // circumcised / penile lesions / urethra normal location, no d/c / testes normal / + cremasteric reflex
FEET + pulses / monofilament + / nails abnormal / dry, broken skin / callus

LABS CBC / CMP / lipids / TSH / microalbumin / A1C / UA, culture / PSA / iron studies / other:

DIAGNOSTICS XR / MRI / CT / US / cardiac / other
REFERRALS   **F/U** ___ wk ___ mo

<table>
<tr><td colspan="2">

Patient ID#:   **Date of visit:**

Reason for visit: **Age:**   **Gender:**

</td><td>

BP: **HT:**
HR: **WT:**
T: **BMI:**
O2%:   **PAIN:**

NOTES . . . .

</td></tr>
</table>

CONST	Δ appetite, energy, weight / fever / chills / sweats / fatigue
HEAD	trauma / mass / tenderness / rash / lesions
EYES	visionΔ / itch / d/c / tears / dry / cataracts / glaucoma / glasses, contacts
ENT	hearing Δ / pain / d/c / vertigo / ? infection // epistaxis / congestion // bleeding, swelling gums / pain / sore throat / voice Δ // neck pain / lumps / swelling / difficulty swallowing
CARDIAC	pain / pressure / dizzy / N / orthopnea / edema / palp / weak w exertion / hx murmurs / hx MI / HTN / HF / numb / tingle / cold extrem / slow wound healing
RESP	wheeze / SOB / cough / asthma / bronch / COPD
GI	abd pain / Δ in bowels / constipation / diarrhea / N V / hepatitis / gallstones / dysphagia / reflux / hemorrhoids / black, bloody stools
GU	burn / pain / nocturia / polyuria / hematuria / incontinence / infection / kid. stones
GENITAL	DC / sores / pain / masses / last pap _____ / sexually active Y N / dyspareunia / LMP _____ / contraception
MSK	redness / swelling / warmth / pain / +/- ROM / arthritis / musc cramps / fracture / sprains / joint replacement / stiffness: AM PM
SKIN	rash / pruritis / jaundice / bruising / hx skin ca / mole Δ / Δ in hair, nails / lesions / slow wound healing
BREASTS	lump / pain / dc / last mammo _____ / self exams YN
NEURO	HA / seizure / vertigo / memory Δ / gait Δ / speech / coord
PSYCH	depression / anxiety / Δ in sleep pattern / substance, ETOH abuse / suicidal ideation / homicidal ideation
ENDO	polydipsia, polyuria / heat, cold intolerance / Δ hair/nails/energy
HEM/LYMPH	anemia / bruising / hx transfusions / blood disorder / lymphadenopathy / axillary, groin tenderness
ALLX/IMMUN	season allx / food allx / med allx / immune disorder:

SOCIAL HX	# in household _____ / lives with SP/BF/GF/SO / children __ / tobacco Y/N #pk / sexual activity Y/N / etoh, other substances Y/N / occupation:
FAM HX	ca / HTN / MI / CAD / stroke / hyperlipidemia / DM2 / Alzheimer's / depression / osteoporosis / other:

GENERAL	well appearing / well nourished / a&o x 3 / normal mood / normal affect
NEURO	intact / abnormal **DTR:** 1 2 3 4 5 location:
SKIN + NAILS	turgor / rash / bruising / lesions // texture, distribution of hair // nails: abnormal color / nail deformity
HEAD	normocephalic / atraumatic / visible mass / palpable mass / depression / scarring
EYES	acuity intact / conjunctiva clear / EOM intact / PERRLA / fundi: normal discs and vessels / icterus / exudate / hemorrhage
EARS	EACs clear / TM translucent, mobile / landmarks abnormal / hearing diminished
NOSE	lesions / mucosal inflammation / septum, turbinates abnormal / sinus tenderness
MOUTH	mucous membranes dry / lesions / poor dentition / caries / gingival inflammation
PHARYNX	mucosa inflammation / tonsillar hypertrophy / tonsillar exudate
NECK	supple / ROM WNL / lesion / bruit / adenopathy / thyroid enlarged, tender / mass
CARDIAC	regular rate, rhythm / S1, S2 / murmur / gallop / click / rub / PMI displacement
RESP	clear to auscultation in all fields / wheezes (insp) (exp) / rales / crackles
ABDOMEN	BSx4 / tender / organomegaly / mass / hernia
RECTAL	abnormal tone / hemorrhoids (int/ext) / palpable mass
BACK	abnormal curvature / tenderness / CVAT / Δ ROM
EXTREMITIES	amputation / deformity / edema / varicosities / + pulses
MSK	abnormal gait / asymmetry / crepitation / defect / tenderness / mass / effusion / Δ ROM / instability / atrophy / abnormal strength, tone in head, neck, spine, ribs, pelvis, UE, LE / pathologic reflexes
PSYCH	A&O x3 / +recent/remote memory / insight / affect
BREAST	nipple abnormality / mass / tenderness / axillary, clavicular adenopathy
GYN/GU	lesions / d/c / uterus, adnexa tenderness / CMT // circumcised / penile lesions / urethra normal location, no d/c / testes normal / + cremasteric reflex
FEET	+ pulses / monofilament + / nails abnormal / dry, broken skin / callus

LABS	CBC / CMP / lipids / TSH / microalbumin / A1C / UA, culture / PSA / iron studies / other:

DIAGNOSTICS	XR / MRI / CT / US / cardiac / other
REFERRALS	**F/U** ___ wk ___ mo

<table>
<tr><td>Patient ID#:</td><td>Date of visit:</td></tr>
<tr><td>Reason for visit:</td><td>Age: Gender:</td></tr>
</table>

BP: HT:
HR: WT:
T: BMI:
O2%:   PAIN:

NOTES . . . .

CONST	Δ appetite, energy, weight / fever / chills / sweats / fatigue
HEAD	trauma / mass / tenderness / rash / lesions
EYES	visionΔ / itch / d/c / tears / dry / cataracts / glaucoma / glasses, contacts
ENT	hearing Δ / pain / d/c / vertigo / ? infection // epistaxis / congestion // bleeding, swelling gums / pain / sore throat / voice Δ // neck pain / lumps / swelling / difficulty swallowing
CARDIAC	pain / pressure / dizzy / N / orthopnea / edema / palp / weak w exertion / hx murmurs / hx MI / HTN / HF / numb / tingle / cold extrem / slow wound healing
RESP	wheeze / SOB / cough / asthma / bronch / COPD
GI	abd pain / Δ in bowels / constipation / diarrhea / N V / hepatitis / gallstones / dysphagia / reflux / hemorrhoids / black, bloody stools
GU	burn / pain / nocturia / polyuria / hematuria / incontinence / infection / kid. stones
GENITAL	DC / sores / pain / masses / last pap _____ / sexually active Y N / dyspareunia / LMP _______ / contraception
MSK	redness / swelling / warmth / pain / +/- ROM / arthritis / musc cramps / fracture / sprains / joint replacement / stiffness: AM PM
SKIN	rash / pruritis / jaundice / bruising / hx skin ca / mole Δ / Δ in hair, nails / lesions / slow wound healing
BREASTS	lump / pain / dc / last mammo _______ / self exams YN
NEURO	HA / seizure / vertigo / memory Δ / gait Δ / speech / coord
PSYCH	depression / anxiety / Δ in sleep pattern / substance, ETOH abuse / suicidal ideation / homicidal ideation
ENDO	polydipsia, polyuria / heat, cold intolerance / Δ hair/nails/energy
HEM/LYMPH	anemia / bruising / hx transfusions / blood disorder / lymphadenopathy / axillary, groin tenderness
ALLX/IMMUN	season allx / food allx / med allx / immune disorder:

SOCIAL HX	# in household _____ / lives with SP/BF/GF/SO / children __ / tobacco Y/N #pk / sexual activity Y/N / etoh, other substances Y/N / occupation:
FAM HX	ca / HTN / MI / CAD / stroke / hyperlipidemia / DM2 / Alzheimer's / depression / osteoporosis / other:

GENERAL	well appearing / well nourished / a&o x 3 / normal mood / normal affect
NEURO	intact / abnormal **DTR:** 1 2 3 4 5 location:
SKIN + NAILS	turgor / rash / bruising / lesions // texture, distribution of hair // nails: abnormal color / nail deformity
HEAD	normocephalic / atraumatic / visible mass / palpable mass / depression / scarring
EYES	acuity intact / conjunctiva clear / EOM intact / PERRLA / fundi: normal discs and vessels / icterus / exudate / hemorrhage
EARS	EACs clear / TM translucent, mobile / landmarks abnormal / hearing diminished
NOSE	lesions / mucosal inflammation / septum, turbinates abnormal / sinus tenderness
MOUTH	mucous membranes dry / lesions / poor dentition / caries / gingival inflammation
PHARYNX	mucosa inflammation / tonsillar hypertrophy / tonsillar exudate
NECK	supple / ROM WNL / lesion / bruit / adenopathy / thyroid enlarged, tender / mass
CARDIAC	regular rate, rhythm / S1, S2 / murmur / gallop / click / rub / PMI displacement
RESP	clear to auscultation in all fields / wheezes (insp) (exp) / rales / crackles
ABDOMEN	BSx4 / tender / organomegaly / mass / hernia
RECTAL	abnormal tone / hemorrhoids (int/ext) / palpable mass
BACK	abnormal curvature / tenderness / CVAT / Δ ROM
EXTREMITIES	amputation / deformity / edema / varicosities / + pulses
MSK	abnormal gait / asymmetry / crepitation / defect / tenderness / mass / effusion / Δ ROM / instability / atrophy / abnormal strength, tone in head, neck, spine, ribs, pelvis, UE, LE / pathologic reflexes
PSYCH	A&O x3 / +recent/remote memory / insight / affect
BREAST	nipple abnormality / mass / tenderness / axillary, clavicular adenopathy
GYN/GU	lesions / d/c / uterus, adnexa tenderness / CMT // circumcised / penile lesions / urethra normal location, no d/c / testes normal / + cremasteric reflex
FEET	+ pulses / monofilament + / nails abnormal / dry, broken skin / callus

LABS	CBC / CMP / lipids / TSH / microalbumin / A1C / UA, culture / PSA / iron studies / other:

DIAGNOSTICS	XR / MRI / CT / US / cardiac / other
REFERRALS	**F/U** ___ wk ___ mo

<table>
<tr><td colspan="2">

Patient ID#:

Reason for visit:
</td><td>

Date of visit:

Age: **Gender:**
</td></tr>
</table>

BP:	**HT:**
HR:	**WT:**
T:	**BMI:**
O2%:	**PAIN:**

NOTES . . . .

CONST Δ appetite, energy, weight / fever / chills / sweats / fatigue
HEAD trauma / mass / tenderness / rash / lesions
EYES visionΔ / itch / d/c / tears / dry / cataracts / glaucoma / glasses, contacts
ENT hearing Δ / pain / d/c / vertigo / ? infection // epistaxis / congestion // bleeding, swelling gums / pain / sore throat / voice Δ // neck pain / lumps / swelling / difficulty swallowing
CARDIAC pain / pressure / dizzy / N / orthopnea / edema / palp / weak w exertion / hx murmurs / hx MI / HTN / HF / numb / tingle / cold extrem / slow wound healing
RESP wheeze / SOB / cough / asthma / bronch / COPD
GI abd pain / Δ in bowels / constipation / diarrhea / N V / hepatitis / gallstones / dysphagia / reflux / hemorrhoids / black, bloody stools
GU burn / pain / nocturia / polyuria / hematuria / incontinence / infection / kid. stones
GENITAL DC / sores / pain / masses / last pap ______ / sexually active Y N / dyspareunia / LMP ______ / contraception
MSK redness / swelling / warmth / pain / +/- ROM / arthritis / musc cramps / fracture / sprains / joint replacement / stiffness: AM PM
SKIN rash / pruritis / jaundice / bruising / hx skin ca / mole Δ / Δ in hair, nails / lesions / slow wound healing
BREASTS lump / pain / dc / last mammo ______ / self exams YN
NEURO HA / seizure / vertigo / memory Δ / gait Δ / speech / coord
PSYCH depression / anxiety / Δ in sleep pattern / substance, ETOH abuse / suicidal ideation / homicidal ideation
ENDO polydipsia, polyuria / heat, cold intolerance / Δ hair/nails/energy
HEM/LYMPH anemia / bruising / hx transfusions / blood disorder / lymphadenopathy / axillary, groin tenderness
ALLX/IMMUN season allx / food allx / med allx / immune disorder:

SOCIAL HX # in household ______ / lives with SP/BF/GF/SO / children __ / tobacco Y/N #pk / sexual activity Y/N / etoh, other substances Y/N / occupation:
FAM HX ca / HTN / MI / CAD / stroke / hyperlipidemia / DM2 / Alzheimer's / depression / osteoporosis / other:

GENERAL well appearing / well nourished / a&o x 3 / normal mood / normal affect
NEURO intact / abnormal   **DTR:** 1 2 3 4 5 location:
SKIN + NAILS turgor / rash / bruising / lesions // texture, distribution of hair // nails: abnormal color / nail deformity
HEAD normocephalic / atraumatic / visible mass / palpable mass / depression / scarring
EYES acuity intact / conjunctiva clear / EOM intact / PERRLA / fundi: normal discs and vessels / icterus / exudate / hemorrhage
EARS EACs clear / TM translucent, mobile / landmarks abnormal / hearing diminished
NOSE lesions / mucosal inflammation / septum, turbinates abnormal / sinus tenderness
MOUTH mucous membranes dry / lesions / poor dentition / caries / gingival inflammation
PHARYNX mucosa inflammation / tonsillar hypertrophy / tonsillar exudate
NECK supple / ROM WNL / lesion / bruit / adenopathy / thyroid enlarged, tender / mass
CARDIAC regular rate, rhythm / S1, S2 / murmur / gallop / click / rub / PMI displacement
RESP clear to auscultation in all fields / wheezes (insp) (exp) / rales / crackles
ABDOMEN BSx4 / tender / organomegaly / mass / hernia
RECTAL abnormal tone / hemorrhoids (int/ext) / palpable mass
BACK abnormal curvature / tenderness / CVAT / Δ ROM
EXTREMITIES amputation / deformity / edema / varicosities / + pulses
MSK abnormal gait / asymmetry / crepitation / defect / tenderness / mass / effusion / Δ ROM / instability / atrophy / abnormal strength, tone in head, neck, spine, ribs, pelvis, UE, LE / pathologic reflexes
PSYCH A&O x3 / +recent/remote memory / insight / affect
BREAST nipple abnormality / mass / tenderness / axillary, clavicular adenopathy
GYN/GU lesions / d/c / uterus, adnexa tenderness / CMT // circumcised / penile lesions / urethra normal location, no d/c / testes normal / + cremasteric reflex
FEET + pulses / monofilament + / nails abnormal / dry, broken skin / callus

---

LABS CBC / CMP / lipids / TSH / microalbumin / A1C / UA, culture / PSA / iron studies / other:

DIAGNOSTICS XR / MRI / CT / US / cardiac / other
REFERRALS   **F/U** ___ wk ___ mo

Patient ID#:	Date of visit:
Reason for visit:	Age: Gender:

BP:	HT:
HR:	WT:
T:	BMI:
O2%:	PAIN:

NOTES . . . .

CONST Δ appetite, energy, weight / fever / chills / sweats / fatigue
HEAD trauma / mass / tenderness / rash / lesions
EYES visionΔ / itch / d/c / tears / dry / cataracts / glaucoma / glasses, contacts
ENT hearing Δ / pain / d/c / vertigo / ? infection // epistaxis / congestion // bleeding, swelling gums / pain / sore throat / voice Δ // neck pain / lumps / swelling / difficulty swallowing

CARDIAC pain / pressure / dizzy / N / orthopnea / edema / palp / weak w exertion / hx murmurs / hx MI / HTN / HF / numb / tingle / cold extrem / slow wound healing

RESP wheeze / SOB / cough / asthma / bronch / COPD
GI abd pain / Δ in bowels / constipation / diarrhea / N V / hepatitis / gallstones / dysphagia / reflux / hemorrhoids / black, bloody stools

GU burn / pain / nocturia / polyuria / hematuria / incontinence / infection / kid. stones
GENITAL DC / sores / pain / masses / last pap ______ / sexually active Y N / dyspareunia / LMP ______ / contraception

MSK redness / swelling / warmth / pain / +/- ROM / arthritis / musc cramps / fracture / sprains / joint replacement / stiffness: AM PM

SKIN rash / pruritis / jaundice / bruising / hx skin ca / mole Δ / Δ in hair, nails / lesions / slow wound healing

BREASTS lump / pain / dc / last mammo ______ / self exams YN
NEURO HA / seizure / vertigo / memory Δ / gait Δ / speech / coord
PSYCH depression / anxiety / Δ in sleep pattern / substance, ETOH abuse / suicidal ideation / homicidal ideation

ENDO polydipsia, polyuria / heat, cold intolerance / Δ hair/nails/energy
HEM/LYMPH anemia / bruising / hx transfusions / blood disorder / lymphadenopathy / axillary, groin tenderness

ALLX/IMMUN season allx / food allx / med allx / immune disorder:

SOCIAL HX # in household ______ / lives with SP/BF/GF/SO / children __ / tobacco Y/N #pk / sexual activity Y/N / etoh, other substances Y/N / occupation:
FAM HX ca / HTN / MI / CAD / stroke / hyperlipidemia / DM2 / Alzheimer's / depression / osteoporosis / other:

GENERAL well appearing / well nourished / a&o x 3 / normal mood / normal affect
NEURO intact / abnormal   **DTR:** 1 2 3 4 5 location:
SKIN + NAILS turgor / rash / bruising / lesions // texture, distribution of hair // nails: abnormal color / nail deformity

HEAD normocephalic / atraumatic / visible mass / palpable mass / depression / scarring
EYES acuity intact / conjunctiva clear / EOM intact / PERRLA / fundi: normal discs and vessels / icterus / exudate / hemorrhage

EARS EACs clear / TM translucent, mobile / landmarks abnormal / hearing diminished
NOSE lesions / mucosal inflammation / septum, turbinates abnormal / sinus tenderness
MOUTH mucous membranes dry / lesions / poor dentition / caries / gingival inflammation
PHARYNX mucosa inflammation / tonsillar hypertrophy / tonsillar exudate
NECK supple / ROM WNL / lesion / bruit / adenopathy / thyroid enlarged, tender / mass
CARDIAC regular rate, rhythm / S1, S2 / murmur / gallop / click / rub / PMI displacement
RESP clear to auscultation in all fields / wheezes (insp) (exp) / rales / crackles
ABDOMEN BSx4 / tender / organomegaly / mass / hernia
RECTAL abnormal tone / hemorrhoids (int/ext) / palpable mass
BACK abnormal curvature / tenderness / CVAT / Δ ROM
EXTREMITIES amputation / deformity / edema / varicosities / + pulses
MSK abnormal gait / asymmetry / crepitation / defect / tenderness / mass / effusion / Δ ROM / instability / atrophy / abnormal strength, tone in head, neck, spine, ribs, pelvis, UE, LE / pathologic reflexes

PSYCH A&O x3 / +recent/remote memory / insight / affect
BREAST nipple abnormality / mass / tenderness / axillary, clavicular adenopathy
GYN/GU lesions / d/c / uterus, adnexa tenderness / CMT // circumcised / penile lesions / urethra normal location, no d/c / testes normal / + cremasteric reflex

FEET + pulses / monofilament + / nails abnormal / dry, broken skin / callus

---

LABS CBC / CMP / lipids / TSH / microalbumin / A1C / UA, culture / PSA / iron studies / other:

DIAGNOSTICS XR / MRI / CT / US / cardiac / other
REFERRALS **F/U** ___ wk ___ mo

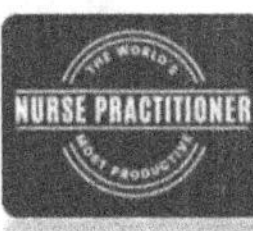

| Patient ID#: | Date of visit: | | BP: | HT: |
| Reason for visit: | Age: Gender: | | HR: | WT: |

BP: HT:
HR: WT:
T: BMI:
O2%:   PAIN:

NOTES . . . .

CONST Δ appetite, energy, weight / fever / chills / sweats / fatigue

HEAD trauma / mass / tenderness / rash / lesions

EYES visionΔ / itch / d/c / tears / dry / cataracts / glaucoma / glasses, contacts

ENT hearing Δ / pain / d/c / vertigo / ? infection // epistaxis / congestion // bleeding, swelling gums / pain / sore throat / voice Δ // neck pain / lumps / swelling / difficulty swallowing

CARDIAC pain / pressure / dizzy / N / orthopnea / edema / palp / weak w exertion / hx murmurs / hx MI / HTN / HF / numb / tingle / cold extrem / slow wound healing

RESP wheeze / SOB / cough / asthma / bronch / COPD

GI abd pain / Δ in bowels / constipation / diarrhea / N V / hepatitis / gallstones / dysphagia / reflux / hemorrhoids / black, bloody stools

GU burn / pain / nocturia / polyuria / hematuria / incontinence / infection / kid. stones

GENITAL DC / sores / pain / masses / last pap ______ / sexually active Y N / dyspareunia / LMP   / contraception

MSK redness / swelling / warmth / pain / +/- ROM / arthritis / musc cramps / fracture / sprains / joint replacement / stiffness: AM PM

SKIN rash / pruritis / jaundice / bruising / hx skin ca / mole Δ / Δ in hair, nails / lesions / slow wound healing

BREASTS lump / pain / dc / last mammo   / self exams YN

NEURO HA / seizure / vertigo / memory Δ / gait Δ / speech / coord

PSYCH depression / anxiety / Δ in sleep pattern / substance, ETOH abuse / suicidal ideation / homicidal ideation

ENDO polydipsia, polyuria / heat, cold intolerance / Δ hair/nails/energy

HEM/LYMPH anemia / bruising / hx transfusions / blood disorder / lymphadenopathy / axillary, groin tenderness

ALLX/IMMUN season allx / food allx / med allx / immune disorder:

SOCIAL HX # in household ______ / lives with SP/BF/GF/SO / children __ / tobacco Y/N #pk / sexual activity Y/N / etoh, other substances Y/N / occupation:

FAM HX ca / HTN / MI / CAD / stroke / hyperlipidemia / DM2 / Alzheimer's / depression / osteoporosis / other:

GENERAL well appearing / well nourished / a&o x 3 / normal mood / normal affect

NEURO intact / abnormal   **DTR:** 1 2 3 4 5 location:

SKIN + NAILS turgor / rash / bruising / lesions // texture, distribution of hair // nails: abnormal color / nail deformity

HEAD normocephalic / atraumatic / visible mass / palpable mass / depression / scarring

EYES acuity intact / conjunctiva clear / EOM intact / PERRLA / fundi: normal discs and vessels / icterus / exudate / hemorrhage

EARS EACs clear / TM translucent, mobile / landmarks abnormal / hearing diminished

NOSE lesions / mucosal inflammation / septum, turbinates abnormal / sinus tenderness

MOUTH mucous membranes dry / lesions / poor dentition / caries / gingival inflammation

PHARYNX mucosa inflammation / tonsillar hypertrophy / tonsillar exudate

NECK supple / ROM WNL / lesion / bruit / adenopathy / thyroid enlarged, tender / mass

CARDIAC regular rate, rhythm / S1, S2 / murmur / gallop / click / rub / PMI displacement

RESP clear to auscultation in all fields / wheezes (insp) (exp) / rales / crackles

ABDOMEN BSx4 / tender / organomegaly / mass / hernia

RECTAL abnormal tone / hemorrhoids (int/ext) / palpable mass

BACK abnormal curvature / tenderness / CVAT / Δ ROM

EXTREMITIES amputation / deformity / edema / varicosities / + pulses

MSK abnormal gait / asymmetry / crepitation / defect / tenderness / mass / effusion / Δ ROM / instability / atrophy / abnormal strength, tone in head, neck, spine, ribs, pelvis, UE, LE / pathologic reflexes

PSYCH A&O x3 / +recent/remote memory / insight / affect

BREAST nipple abnormality / mass / tenderness / axillary, clavicular adenopathy

GYN/GU lesions / d/c / uterus, adnexa tenderness / CMT // circumcised / penile lesions / urethra normal location, no d/c / testes normal / + cremasteric reflex

FEET + pulses / monofilament + / nails abnormal / dry, broken skin / callus

LABS CBC / CMP / lipids / TSH / microalbumin / A1C / UA, culture / PSA / iron studies / other:

DIAGNOSTICS XR / MRI / CT / US / cardiac / other

REFERRALS   **F/U** ___ wk ___ mo

<table>
<tr><td colspan="2">Patient ID#:
Reason for visit:</td><td>Date of visit:
Age: Gender:</td></tr>
</table>

BP: HT:
HR: WT:
T: BMI:
O2%:   PAIN:

NOTES . . . .

CONST	Δ appetite, energy, weight / fever / chills / sweats / fatigue
HEAD	trauma / mass / tenderness / rash / lesions
EYES	visionΔ / itch / d/c / tears / dry / cataracts / glaucoma / glasses, contacts
ENT	hearing Δ / pain / d/c / vertigo / ? infection // epistaxis / congestion // bleeding, swelling gums / pain / sore throat / voice Δ // neck pain / lumps / swelling / difficulty swallowing
CARDIAC	pain / pressure / dizzy / N / orthopnea / edema / palp / weak w exertion / hx murmurs / hx MI / HTN / HF / numb / tingle / cold extrem / slow wound healing
RESP	wheeze / SOB / cough / asthma / bronch / COPD
GI	abd pain / Δ in bowels / constipation / diarrhea / N V / hepatitis / gallstones / dysphagia / reflux / hemorrhoids / black, bloody stools
GU	burn / pain / nocturia / polyuria / hematuria / incontinence / infection / kid. stones
GENITAL	DC / sores / pain / masses / last pap _____ / sexually active Y N / dyspareunia / LMP / contraception
MSK	redness / swelling / warmth / pain / +/- ROM / arthritis / musc cramps / fracture / sprains / joint replacement / stiffness: AM PM
SKIN	rash / pruritis / jaundice / bruising / hx skin ca / mole Δ / Δ in hair, nails / lesions / slow wound healing
BREASTS	lump / pain / dc / last mammo / self exams YN
NEURO	HA / seizure / vertigo / memory Δ / gait Δ / speech / coord
PSYCH	depression / anxiety / Δ in sleep pattern / substance, ETOH abuse / suicidal ideation / homicidal ideation
ENDO	polydipsia, polyuria / heat, cold intolerance / Δ hair/nails/energy
HEM/LYMPH	anemia / bruising / hx transfusions / blood disorder / lymphadenopathy / axillary, groin tenderness
ALLX/IMMUN	season allx / food allx / med allx / immune disorder:

SOCIAL HX	# in household _____ / lives with SP/BF/GF/SO / children __ / tobacco Y/N #pk / sexual activity Y/N / etoh, other substances Y/N / occupation:
FAM HX	ca / HTN / MI / CAD / stroke / hyperlipidemia / DM2 / Alzheimer's / depression / osteoporosis / other:

GENERAL	well appearing / well nourished / a&o x 3 / normal mood / normal affect
NEURO	intact / abnormal **DTR:** 1 2 3 4 5 location:
SKIN + NAILS	turgor / rash / bruising / lesions // texture, distribution of hair // nails: abnormal color / nail deformity
HEAD	normocephalic / atraumatic / visible mass / palpable mass / depression / scarring
EYES	acuity intact / conjunctiva clear / EOM intact / PERRLA / fundi: normal discs and vessels / icterus / exudate / hemorrhage
EARS	EACs clear / TM translucent, mobile / landmarks abnormal / hearing diminished
NOSE	lesions / mucosal inflammation / septum, turbinates abnormal / sinus tenderness
MOUTH	mucous membranes dry / lesions / poor dentition / caries / gingival inflammation
PHARYNX	mucosa inflammation / tonsillar hypertrophy / tonsillar exudate
NECK	supple / ROM WNL / lesion / bruit / adenopathy / thyroid enlarged, tender / mass
CARDIAC	regular rate, rhythm / S1, S2 / murmur / gallop / click / rub / PMI displacement
RESP	clear to auscultation in all fields / wheezes (insp) (exp) / rales / crackles
ABDOMEN	BSx4 / tender / organomegaly / mass / hernia
RECTAL	abnormal tone / hemorrhoids (int/ext) / palpable mass
BACK	abnormal curvature / tenderness / CVAT / Δ ROM
EXTREMITIES	amputation / deformity / edema / varicosities / + pulses
MSK	abnormal gait / asymmetry / crepitation / defect / tenderness / mass / effusion / Δ ROM / instability / atrophy / abnormal strength, tone in head, neck, spine, ribs, pelvis, UE, LE / pathologic reflexes
PSYCH	A&O x3 / +recent/remote memory / insight / affect
BREAST	nipple abnormality / mass / tenderness / axillary, clavicular adenopathy
GYN/GU	lesions / d/c / uterus, adnexa tenderness / CMT // circumcised / penile lesions / urethra normal location, no d/c / testes normal / + cremasteric reflex
FEET	+ pulses / monofilament + / nails abnormal / dry, broken skin / callus

LABS	CBC / CMP / lipids / TSH / microalbumin / A1C / UA, culture / PSA / iron studies / other:

DIAGNOSTICS	XR / MRI / CT / US / cardiac / other
REFERRALS	**F/U** ___ wk ___ mo

<table>
<tr><td colspan="2">

Patient ID#:
Reason for visit:
</td><td>

Date of visit:
Age: **Gender:**
</td></tr>
</table>

<table>
<tr><td>

BP:
</td><td>

HT:
</td></tr>
<tr><td>

HR:
</td><td>

WT:
</td></tr>
<tr><td>

T:
</td><td>

BMI:
</td></tr>
<tr><td>

O2%:
</td><td>

PAIN:
</td></tr>
</table>

NOTES . . . .

CONST	Δ appetite, energy, weight / fever / chills / sweats / fatigue
HEAD	trauma / mass / tenderness / rash / lesions
EYES	visionΔ / itch / d/c / tears / dry / cataracts / glaucoma / glasses, contacts
ENT	hearing Δ / pain / d/c / vertigo / ? infection // epistaxis / congestion // bleeding, swelling gums / pain / sore throat / voice Δ // neck pain / lumps / swelling / difficulty swallowing
CARDIAC	pain / pressure / dizzy / N / orthopnea / edema / palp / weak w exertion / hx murmurs / hx MI / HTN / HF / numb / tingle / cold extrem / slow wound healing
RESP	wheeze / SOB / cough / asthma / bronch / COPD
GI	abd pain / Δ in bowels / constipation / diarrhea / N V / hepatitis / gallstones / dysphagia / reflux / hemorrhoids / black, bloody stools
GU	burn / pain / nocturia / polyuria / hematuria / incontinence / infection / kid. stones
GENITAL	DC / sores / pain / masses / last pap ______ / sexually active Y N / dyspareunia / LMP ______ / contraception
MSK	redness / swelling / warmth / pain / +/- ROM / arthritis / musc cramps / fracture / sprains / joint replacement / stiffness: AM PM
SKIN	rash / pruritis / jaundice / bruising / hx skin ca / mole Δ / Δ in hair, nails / lesions / slow wound healing
BREASTS	lump / pain / dc / last mammo ______ / self exams YN
NEURO	HA / seizure / vertigo / memory Δ / gait Δ / speech / coord
PSYCH	depression / anxiety / Δ in sleep pattern / substance, ETOH abuse / suicidal ideation / homicidal ideation
ENDO	polydipsia, polyuria / heat, cold intolerance / Δ hair/nails/energy
HEM/LYMPH	anemia / bruising / hx transfusions / blood disorder / lymphadenopathy / axillary, groin tenderness
ALLX/IMMUN	season allx / food allx / med allx / immune disorder:

SOCIAL HX	# in household ______ / lives with SP/BF/GF/SO / children __ / tobacco Y/N #pk / sexual activity Y/N / etoh, other substances Y/N / occupation:
FAM HX	ca / HTN / MI / CAD / stroke / hyperlipidemia / DM2 / Alzheimer's / depression / osteoporosis / other:

GENERAL	well appearing / well nourished / a&o x 3 / normal mood / normal affect
NEURO	intact / abnormal **DTR:** 1 2 3 4 5 location:
SKIN + NAILS	turgor / rash / bruising / lesions // texture, distribution of hair // nails: abnormal color / nail deformity
HEAD	normocephalic / atraumatic / visible mass / palpable mass / depression / scarring
EYES	acuity intact / conjunctiva clear / EOM intact / PERRLA / fundi: normal discs and vessels / icterus / exudate / hemorrhage
EARS	EACs clear / TM translucent, mobile / landmarks abnormal / hearing diminished
NOSE	lesions / mucosal inflammation / septum, turbinates abnormal / sinus tenderness
MOUTH	mucous membranes dry / lesions / poor dentition / caries / gingival inflammation
PHARYNX	mucosa inflammation / tonsillar hypertrophy / tonsillar exudate
NECK	supple / ROM WNL / lesion / bruit / adenopathy / thyroid enlarged, tender / mass
CARDIAC	regular rate, rhythm / S1, S2 / murmur / gallop / click / rub / PMI displacement
RESP	clear to auscultation in all fields / wheezes (insp) (exp) / rales / crackles
ABDOMEN	BSx4 / tender / organomegaly / mass / hernia
RECTAL	abnormal tone / hemorrhoids (int/ext) / palpable mass
BACK	abnormal curvature / tenderness / CVAT / Δ ROM
EXTREMITIES	amputation / deformity / edema / varicosities / + pulses
MSK	abnormal gait / asymmetry / crepitation / defect / tenderness / mass / effusion / Δ ROM / instability / atrophy / abnormal strength, tone in head, neck, spine, ribs, pelvis, UE, LE / pathologic reflexes
PSYCH	A&O x3 / +recent/remote memory / insight / affect
BREAST	nipple abnormality / mass / tenderness / axillary, clavicular adenopathy
GYN/GU	lesions / d/c / uterus, adnexa tenderness / CMT // circumcised / penile lesions / urethra normal location, no d/c / testes normal / + cremasteric reflex
FEET	+ pulses / monofilament + / nails abnormal / dry, broken skin / callus

LABS	CBC / CMP / lipids / TSH / microalbumin / A1C / UA, culture / PSA / iron studies / other:

DIAGNOSTICS	XR / MRI / CT / US / cardiac / other
REFERRALS	**F/U** ___ wk ___ mo

<table>
<tr><td>Patient ID#:</td><td>Date of visit:</td></tr>
<tr><td>Reason for visit:</td><td>Age: Gender:</td></tr>
</table>

BP:	HT:
HR:	WT:
T:	BMI:
O2%:	PAIN:

NOTES . . . .

CONST	Δ appetite, energy, weight / fever / chills / sweats / fatigue
HEAD	trauma / mass / tenderness / rash / lesions
EYES	visionΔ / itch / d/c / tears / dry / cataracts / glaucoma / glasses, contacts
ENT	hearing Δ / pain / d/c / vertigo / ? infection // epistaxis / congestion // bleeding, swelling gums / pain / sore throat / voice Δ // neck pain / lumps / swelling / difficulty swallowing
CARDIAC	pain / pressure / dizzy / N / orthopnea / edema / palp / weak w exertion / hx murmurs / hx MI / HTN / HF / numb / tingle / cold extrem / slow wound healing
RESP	wheeze / SOB / cough / asthma / bronch / COPD
GI	abd pain / Δ in bowels / constipation / diarrhea / N V / hepatitis / gallstones / dysphagia / reflux / hemorrhoids / black, bloody stools
GU	burn / pain / nocturia / polyuria / hematuria / incontinence / infection / kid. stones
GENITAL	DC / sores / pain / masses / last pap ______ / sexually active Y N / dyspareunia / LMP / contraception
MSK	redness / swelling / warmth / pain / +/- ROM / arthritis / musc cramps / fracture / sprains / joint replacement / stiffness: AM PM
SKIN	rash / pruritis / jaundice / bruising / hx skin ca / mole Δ / Δ in hair, nails / lesions / slow wound healing
BREASTS	lump / pain / dc / last mammo ______ / self exams YN
NEURO	HA / seizure / vertigo / memory Δ / gait Δ / speech / coord
PSYCH	depression / anxiety / Δ in sleep pattern / substance, ETOH abuse / suicidal ideation / homicidal ideation
ENDO	polydipsia, polyuria / heat, cold intolerance / Δ hair/nails/energy
HEM/LYMPH	anemia / bruising / hx transfusions / blood disorder / lymphadenopathy / axillary, groin tenderness
ALLX/IMMUN	season allx / food allx / med allx / immune disorder:

SOCIAL HX	# in household ______ / lives with SP/BF/GF/SO / children __ / tobacco Y/N #pk / sexual activity Y/N / etoh, other substances Y/N / occupation:
FAM HX	ca / HTN / MI / CAD / stroke / hyperlipidemia / DM2 / Alzheimer's / depression / osteoporosis / other:

GENERAL	well appearing / well nourished / a&o x 3 / normal mood / normal affect
NEURO	intact / abnormal **DTR:** 1 2 3 4 5 location:
SKIN + NAILS	turgor / rash / bruising / lesions // texture, distribution of hair // nails: abnormal color / nail deformity
HEAD	normocephalic / atraumatic / visible mass / palpable mass / depression / scarring
EYES	acuity intact / conjunctiva clear / EOM intact / PERRLA / fundi: normal discs and vessels / icterus / exudate / hemorrhage
EARS	EACs clear / TM translucent, mobile / landmarks abnormal / hearing diminished
NOSE	lesions / mucosal inflammation / septum, turbinates abnormal / sinus tenderness
MOUTH	mucous membranes dry / lesions / poor dentition / caries / gingival inflammation
PHARYNX	mucosa inflammation / tonsillar hypertrophy / tonsillar exudate
NECK	supple / ROM WNL / lesion / bruit / adenopathy / thyroid enlarged, tender / mass
CARDIAC	regular rate, rhythm / S1, S2 / murmur / gallop / click / rub / PMI displacement
RESP	clear to auscultation in all fields / wheezes (insp) (exp) / rales / crackles
ABDOMEN	BSx4 / tender / organomegaly / mass / hernia
RECTAL	abnormal tone / hemorrhoids (int/ext) / palpable mass
BACK	abnormal curvature / tenderness / CVAT / Δ ROM
EXTREMITIES	amputation / deformity / edema / varicosities / + pulses
MSK	abnormal gait / asymmetry / crepitation / defect / tenderness / mass / effusion / Δ ROM / instability / atrophy / abnormal strength, tone in head, neck, spine, ribs, pelvis, UE, LE / pathologic reflexes
PSYCH	A&O x3 / +recent/remote memory / insight / affect
BREAST	nipple abnormality / mass / tenderness / axillary, clavicular adenopathy
GYN/GU	lesions / d/c / uterus, adnexa tenderness / CMT // circumcised / penile lesions / urethra normal location, no d/c / testes normal / + cremasteric reflex
FEET	+ pulses / monofilament + / nails abnormal / dry, broken skin / callus

LABS	CBC / CMP / lipids / TSH / microalbumin / A1C / UA, culture / PSA / iron studies / other:

DIAGNOSTICS	XR / MRI / CT / US / cardiac / other
REFERRALS	**F/U** ___ wk ___ mo

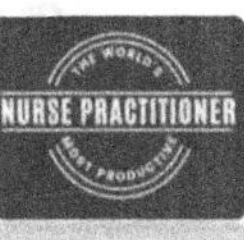

<table>
<tr><td colspan="2">

Patient ID#:   **Date of visit:**

Reason for visit: **Age:**   **Gender:**

</td><td>

BP: **HT:**
HR: **WT:**
T: **BMI:**
O2%:   **PAIN:**

</td></tr>
</table>

NOTES . . . .

CONST	Δ appetite, energy, weight / fever / chills / sweats / fatigue
HEAD	trauma / mass / tenderness / rash / lesions
EYES	visionΔ / itch / d/c / tears / dry / cataracts / glaucoma / glasses, contacts
ENT	hearing Δ / pain / d/c / vertigo / ? infection // epistaxis / congestion // bleeding, swelling gums / pain / sore throat / voice Δ // neck pain / lumps / swelling / difficulty swallowing
CARDIAC	pain / pressure / dizzy / N / orthopnea / edema / palp / weak w exertion / hx murmurs / hx MI / HTN / HF / numb / tingle / cold extrem / slow wound healing
RESP	wheeze / SOB / cough / asthma / bronch / COPD
GI	abd pain / Δ in bowels / constipation / diarrhea / N V / hepatitis / gallstones / dysphagia / reflux / hemorrhoids / black, bloody stools
GU	burn / pain / nocturia / polyuria / hematuria / incontinence / infection / kid. stones
GENITAL	DC / sores / pain / masses / last pap ______ / sexually active Y N / dyspareunia / LMP ______ / contraception
MSK	redness / swelling / warmth / pain / +/- ROM / arthritis / musc cramps / fracture / sprains / joint replacement / stiffness: AM PM
SKIN	rash / pruritis / jaundice / bruising / hx skin ca / mole Δ / Δ in hair, nails / lesions / slow wound healing
BREASTS	lump / pain / dc / last mammo ______ / self exams YN
NEURO	HA / seizure / vertigo / memory Δ / gait Δ / speech / coord
PSYCH	depression / anxiety / Δ in sleep pattern / substance, ETOH abuse / suicidal ideation / homicidal ideation
ENDO	polydipsia, polyuria / heat, cold intolerance / Δ hair/nails/energy
HEM/LYMPH	anemia / bruising / hx transfusions / blood disorder / lymphadenopathy / axillary, groin tenderness
ALLX/IMMUN	season allx / food allx / med allx / immune disorder:

SOCIAL HX	# in household ______ / lives with SP/BF/GF/SO / children __ / tobacco Y/N #pk / sexual activity Y/N / etoh, other substances Y/N / occupation:
FAM HX	ca / HTN / MI / CAD / stroke / hyperlipidemia / DM2 / Alzheimer's / depression / osteoporosis / other:

GENERAL	well appearing / well nourished / a&o x 3 / normal mood / normal affect
NEURO	intact / abnormal **DTR:** 1 2 3 4 5 location:
SKIN + NAILS	turgor / rash / bruising / lesions // texture, distribution of hair // nails: abnormal color / nail deformity
HEAD	normocephalic / atraumatic / visible mass / palpable mass / depression / scarring
EYES	acuity intact / conjunctiva clear / EOM intact / PERRLA / fundi: normal discs and vessels / icterus / exudate / hemorrhage
EARS	EACs clear / TM translucent, mobile / landmarks abnormal / hearing diminished
NOSE	lesions / mucosal inflammation / septum, turbinates abnormal / sinus tenderness
MOUTH	mucous membranes dry / lesions / poor dentition / caries / gingival inflammation
PHARYNX	mucosa inflammation / tonsillar hypertrophy / tonsillar exudate
NECK	supple / ROM WNL / lesion / bruit / adenopathy / thyroid enlarged, tender / mass
CARDIAC	regular rate, rhythm / S1, S2 / murmur / gallop / click / rub / PMI displacement
RESP	clear to auscultation in all fields / wheezes (insp) (exp) / rales / crackles
ABDOMEN	BSx4 / tender / organomegaly / mass / hernia
RECTAL	abnormal tone / hemorrhoids (int/ext) / palpable mass
BACK	abnormal curvature / tenderness / CVAT / Δ ROM
EXTREMITIES	amputation / deformity / edema / varicosities / + pulses
MSK	abnormal gait / asymmetry / crepitation / defect / tenderness / mass / effusion / Δ ROM / instability / atrophy / abnormal strength, tone in head, neck, spine, ribs, pelvis, UE, LE / pathologic reflexes
PSYCH	A&O x3 / +recent/remote memory / insight / affect
BREAST	nipple abnormality / mass / tenderness / axillary, clavicular adenopathy
GYN/GU	lesions / d/c / uterus, adnexa tenderness / CMT // circumcised / penile lesions / urethra normal location, no d/c / testes normal / + cremasteric reflex
FEET	+ pulses / monofilament + / nails abnormal / dry, broken skin / callus

LABS	CBC / CMP / lipids / TSH / microalbumin / A1C / UA, culture / PSA / iron studies / other:

DIAGNOSTICS	XR / MRI / CT / US / cardiac / other
REFERRALS	**F/U** ___ wk ___ mo

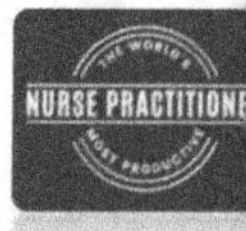

<table>
<tr><td colspan="2">Patient ID#:
Reason for visit:</td><td>Date of visit:
Age: Gender:</td></tr>
</table>

BP:	**HT:**
HR:	**WT:**
T:	**BMI:**
O2%:	**PAIN:**

NOTES . . . .

CONST Δ appetite, energy, weight / fever / chills / sweats / fatigue
HEAD trauma / mass / tenderness / rash / lesions
EYES visionΔ / itch / d/c / tears / dry / cataracts / glaucoma / glasses, contacts
ENT hearing Δ / pain / d/c / vertigo / ? infection // epistaxis / congestion // bleeding, swelling gums / pain / sore throat / voice Δ // neck pain / lumps / swelling / difficulty swallowing

CARDIAC pain / pressure / dizzy / N / orthopnea / edema / palp / weak w exertion / hx murmurs / hx MI / HTN / HF / numb / tingle / cold extrem / slow wound healing

RESP wheeze / SOB / cough / asthma / bronch / COPD
GI abd pain / Δ in bowels / constipation / diarrhea / N V / hepatitis / gallstones / dysphagia / reflux / hemorrhoids / black, bloody stools

GU burn / pain / nocturia / polyuria / hematuria / incontinence / infection / kid. stones
GENITAL DC / sores / pain / masses / last pap ______ / sexually active Y N / dyspareunia / LMP ________ / contraception

MSK redness / swelling / warmth / pain / +/- ROM / arthritis / musc cramps / fracture / sprains / joint replacement / stiffness: AM PM
SKIN rash / pruritis / jaundice / bruising / hx skin ca / mole Δ / Δ in hair, nails / lesions / slow wound healing

BREASTS lump / pain / dc / last mammo ________ / self exams YN
NEURO HA / seizure / vertigo / memory Δ / gait Δ / speech / coord
PSYCH depression / anxiety / Δ in sleep pattern / substance, ETOH abuse / suicidal ideation / homicidal ideation

ENDO polydipsia, polyuria / heat, cold intolerance / Δ hair/nails/energy
HEM/LYMPH anemia / bruising / hx transfusions / blood disorder / lymphadenopathy / axillary, groin tenderness

ALLX/IMMUN season allx / food allx / med allx / immune disorder:

SOCIAL HX # in household ______ / lives with SP/BF/GF/SO / children __ / tobacco Y/N #pk / sexual activity Y/N / etoh, other substances Y/N / occupation:
FAM HX ca / HTN / MI / CAD / stroke / hyperlipidemia / DM2 / Alzheimer's / depression / osteoporosis / other:

GENERAL well appearing / well nourished / a&o x 3 / normal mood / normal affect
NEURO intact / abnormal   **DTR:** 1 2 3 4 5 location:
SKIN + NAILS turgor / rash / bruising / lesions // texture, distribution of hair // nails: abnormal color / nail deformity

HEAD normocephalic / atraumatic / visible mass / palpable mass / depression / scarring
EYES acuity intact / conjunctiva clear / EOM intact / PERRLA / fundi: normal discs and vessels / icterus / exudate / hemorrhage

EARS EACs clear / TM translucent, mobile / landmarks abnormal / hearing diminished
NOSE lesions / mucosal inflammation / septum, turbinates abnormal / sinus tenderness
MOUTH mucous membranes dry / lesions / poor dentition / caries / gingival inflammation
PHARYNX mucosa inflammation / tonsillar hypertrophy / tonsillar exudate
NECK supple / ROM WNL / lesion / bruit / adenopathy / thyroid enlarged, tender / mass
CARDIAC regular rate, rhythm / S1, S2 / murmur / gallop / click / rub / PMI displacement
RESP clear to auscultation in all fields / wheezes (insp) (exp) / rales / crackles
ABDOMEN BSx4 / tender / organomegaly / mass / hernia
RECTAL abnormal tone / hemorrhoids (int/ext) / palpable mass
BACK abnormal curvature / tenderness / CVAT / Δ ROM
EXTREMITIES amputation / deformity / edema / varicosities / + pulses
MSK abnormal gait / asymmetry / crepitation / defect / tenderness / mass / effusion / Δ ROM / instability / atrophy / abnormal strength, tone in head, neck, spine, ribs, pelvis, UE, LE / pathologic reflexes

PSYCH A&O x3 / +recent/remote memory / insight / affect
BREAST nipple abnormality / mass / tenderness / axillary, clavicular adenopathy
GYN/GU lesions / d/c / uterus, adnexa tenderness / CMT // circumcised / penile lesions / urethra normal location, no d/c / testes normal / + cremasteric reflex
FEET + pulses / monofilament + / nails abnormal / dry, broken skin / callus

---

LABS CBC / CMP / lipids / TSH / microalbumin / A1C / UA, culture / PSA / iron studies / other:

DIAGNOSTICS XR / MRI / CT / US / cardiac / other
REFERRALS   **F/U** ___ wk ___ mo

<table>
<tr><td>

Patient ID#:

Reason for visit:

</td><td>

Date of visit:

Age: Gender:

</td></tr>
</table>

BP: HT:

HR: WT:

T: BMI:

O2%:   PAIN:

NOTES . . . .

CONST	Δ appetite, energy, weight / fever / chills / sweats / fatigue
HEAD	trauma / mass / tenderness / rash / lesions
EYES	visionΔ / itch / d/c / tears / dry / cataracts / glaucoma / glasses, contacts
ENT	hearing Δ / pain / d/c / vertigo / ? infection // epistaxis / congestion // bleeding, swelling gums / pain / sore throat / voice Δ // neck pain / lumps / swelling / difficulty swallowing
CARDIAC	pain / pressure / dizzy / N / orthopnea / edema / palp / weak w exertion / hx murmurs / hx MI / HTN / HF / numb / tingle / cold extrem / slow wound healing
RESP	wheeze / SOB / cough / asthma / bronch / COPD
GI	abd pain / Δ in bowels / constipation / diarrhea / N V / hepatitis / gallstones / dysphagia / reflux / hemorrhoids / black, bloody stools
GU	burn / pain / nocturia / polyuria / hematuria / incontinence / infection / kid. stones
GENITAL	DC / sores / pain / masses / last pap _____ / sexually active Y N / dyspareunia / LMP _______ / contraception
MSK	redness / swelling / warmth / pain / +/- ROM / arthritis / musc cramps / fracture / sprains / joint replacement / stiffness: AM PM
SKIN	rash / pruritis / jaundice / bruising / hx skin ca / mole Δ / Δ in hair, nails / lesions / slow wound healing
BREASTS	lump / pain / dc / last mammo _____ / self exams YN
NEURO	HA / seizure / vertigo / memory Δ / gait Δ / speech / coord
PSYCH	depression / anxiety / Δ in sleep pattern / substance, ETOH abuse / suicidal ideation / homicidal ideation
ENDO	polydipsia, polyuria / heat, cold intolerance / Δ hair/nails/energy
HEM/LYMPH	anemia / bruising / hx transfusions / blood disorder / lymphadenopathy / axillary, groin tenderness
ALLX/IMMUN	season allx / food allx / med allx / immune disorder:

SOCIAL HX	# in household _______ / lives with SP/BF/GF/SO / children __ / tobacco Y/N #pk / sexual activity Y/N / etoh, other substances Y/N / occupation:
FAM HX	ca / HTN / MI / CAD / stroke / hyperlipidemia / DM2 / Alzheimer's / depression / osteoporosis / other:

GENERAL	well appearing / well nourished / a&o x 3 / normal mood / normal affect
NEURO	intact / abnormal **DTR:** 1 2 3 4 5 location:
SKIN + NAILS	turgor / rash / bruising / lesions // texture, distribution of hair // nails: abnormal color / nail deformity
HEAD	normocephalic / atraumatic / visible mass / palpable mass / depression / scarring
EYES	acuity intact / conjunctiva clear / EOM intact / PERRLA / fundi: normal discs and vessels / icterus / exudate / hemorrhage
EARS	EACs clear / TM translucent, mobile / landmarks abnormal / hearing diminished
NOSE	lesions / mucosal inflammation / septum, turbinates abnormal / sinus tenderness
MOUTH	mucous membranes dry / lesions / poor dentition / caries / gingival inflammation
PHARYNX	mucosa inflammation / tonsillar hypertrophy / tonsillar exudate
NECK	supple / ROM WNL / lesion / bruit / adenopathy / thyroid enlarged, tender / mass
CARDIAC	regular rate, rhythm / S1, S2 / murmur / gallop / click / rub / PMI displacement
RESP	clear to auscultation in all fields / wheezes (insp) (exp) / rales / crackles
ABDOMEN	BSx4 / tender / organomegaly / mass / hernia
RECTAL	abnormal tone / hemorrhoids (int/ext) / palpable mass
BACK	abnormal curvature / tenderness / CVAT / Δ ROM
EXTREMITIES	amputation / deformity / edema / varicosities / + pulses
MSK	abnormal gait / asymmetry / crepitation / defect / tenderness / mass / effusion / Δ ROM / instability / atrophy / abnormal strength, tone in head, neck, spine, ribs, pelvis, UE, LE / pathologic reflexes
PSYCH	A&O x3 / +recent/remote memory / insight / affect
BREAST	nipple abnormality / mass / tenderness / axillary, clavicular adenopathy
GYN/GU	lesions / d/c / uterus, adnexa tenderness / CMT // circumcised / penile lesions / urethra normal location, no d/c / testes normal / + cremasteric reflex
FEET	+ pulses / monofilament + / nails abnormal / dry, broken skin / callus

LABS	CBC / CMP / lipids / TSH / microalbumin / A1C / UA, culture / PSA / iron studies / other:

DIAGNOSTICS	XR / MRI / CT / US / cardiac / other
REFERRALS	**F/U** ___ wk ___ mo

<table>
<tr><td colspan="2">

Patient ID#:

Reason for visit:
</td><td>

Date of visit:

Age: Gender:
</td></tr>
</table>

BP: HT:
HR: WT:
T: BMI:
O2%:   PAIN:

NOTES . . . .

CONST	Δ appetite, energy, weight / fever / chills / sweats / fatigue
HEAD	trauma / mass / tenderness / rash / lesions
EYES	visionΔ / itch / d/c / tears / dry / cataracts / glaucoma / glasses, contacts
ENT	hearing Δ / pain / d/c / vertigo / ? infection // epistaxis / congestion // bleeding, swelling gums / pain / sore throat / voice Δ // neck pain / lumps / swelling / difficulty swallowing
CARDIAC	pain / pressure / dizzy / N / orthopnea / edema / palp / weak w exertion / hx murmurs / hx MI / HTN / HF / numb / tingle / cold extrem / slow wound healing
RESP	wheeze / SOB / cough / asthma / bronch / COPD
GI	abd pain / Δ in bowels / constipation / diarrhea / N V / hepatitis / gallstones / dysphagia / reflux / hemorrhoids / black, bloody stools
GU	burn / pain / nocturia / polyuria / hematuria / incontinence / infection / kid. stones
GENITAL	DC / sores / pain / masses / last pap ______ / sexually active Y N / dyspareunia / LMP ______ / contraception
MSK	redness / swelling / warmth / pain / +/- ROM / arthritis / musc cramps / fracture / sprains / joint replacement / stiffness: AM PM
SKIN	rash / pruritis / jaundice / bruising / hx skin ca / mole Δ / Δ in hair, nails / lesions / slow wound healing
BREASTS	lump / pain / dc / last mammo ______ / self exams YN
NEURO	HA / seizure / vertigo / memory Δ / gait Δ / speech / coord
PSYCH	depression / anxiety / Δ in sleep pattern / substance, ETOH abuse / suicidal ideation / homicidal ideation
ENDO	polydipsia, polyuria / heat, cold intolerance / Δ hair/nails/energy
HEM/LYMPH	anemia / bruising / hx transfusions / blood disorder / lymphadenopathy / axillary, groin tenderness
ALLX/IMMUN	season allx / food allx / med allx / immune disorder:

SOCIAL HX	# in household ______ / lives with SP/BF/GF/SO / children ___ / tobacco Y/N #pk / sexual activity Y/N / etoh, other substances Y/N / occupation:
FAM HX	ca / HTN / MI / CAD / stroke / hyperlipidemia / DM2 / Alzheimer's / depression / osteoporosis / other:

GENERAL	well appearing / well nourished / a&o x 3 / normal mood / normal affect
NEURO	intact / abnormal **DTR:** 1 2 3 4 5 location:
SKIN + NAILS	turgor / rash / bruising / lesions // texture, distribution of hair // nails: abnormal color / nail deformity
HEAD	normocephalic / atraumatic / visible mass / palpable mass / depression / scarring
EYES	acuity intact / conjunctiva clear / EOM intact / PERRLA / fundi: normal discs and vessels / icterus / exudate / hemorrhage
EARS	EACs clear / TM translucent, mobile / landmarks abnormal / hearing diminished
NOSE	lesions / mucosal inflammation / septum, turbinates abnormal / sinus tenderness
MOUTH	mucous membranes dry / lesions / poor dentition / caries / gingival inflammation
PHARYNX	mucosa inflammation / tonsillar hypertrophy / tonsillar exudate
NECK	supple / ROM WNL / lesion / bruit / adenopathy / thyroid enlarged, tender / mass
CARDIAC	regular rate, rhythm / S1, S2 / murmur / gallop / click / rub / PMI displacement
RESP	clear to auscultation in all fields / wheezes (insp) (exp) / rales / crackles
ABDOMEN	BSx4 / tender / organomegaly / mass / hernia
RECTAL	abnormal tone / hemorrhoids (int/ext) / palpable mass
BACK	abnormal curvature / tenderness / CVAT / Δ ROM
EXTREMITIES	amputation / deformity / edema / varicosities / + pulses
MSK	abnormal gait / asymmetry / crepitation / defect / tenderness / mass / effusion / Δ ROM / instability / atrophy / abnormal strength, tone in head, neck, spine, ribs, pelvis, UE, LE / pathologic reflexes
PSYCH	A&O x3 / +recent/remote memory / insight / affect
BREAST	nipple abnormality / mass / tenderness / axillary, clavicular adenopathy
GYN/GU	lesions / d/c / uterus, adnexa tenderness / CMT // circumcised / penile lesions / urethra normal location, no d/c / testes normal / + cremasteric reflex
FEET	+ pulses / monofilament + / nails abnormal / dry, broken skin / callus

LABS	CBC / CMP / lipids / TSH / microalbumin / A1C / UA, culture / PSA / iron studies / other:

DIAGNOSTICS	XR / MRI / CT / US / cardiac / other
REFERRALS	**F/U** ___ wk ___ mo

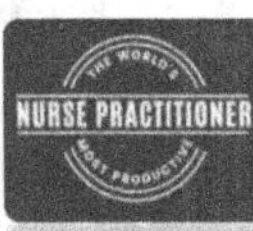

<table>
<tr><td colspan="2">

Patient ID#:   **Date of visit:**
Reason for visit: **Age:**   **Gender:**

</td><td>

BP: **HT:**
HR: **WT:**
T: **BMI:**
O2%:   **PAIN:**

</td></tr>
</table>

NOTES . . . .

CONST	Δ appetite, energy, weight / fever / chills / sweats / fatigue
HEAD	trauma / mass / tenderness / rash / lesions
EYES	visionΔ / itch / d/c / tears / dry / cataracts / glaucoma / glasses, contacts
ENT	hearing Δ / pain / d/c / vertigo / ? infection // epistaxis / congestion // bleeding, swelling gums / pain / sore throat / voice Δ // neck pain / lumps / swelling / difficulty swallowing
CARDIAC	pain / pressure / dizzy / N / orthopnea / edema / palp / weak w exertion / hx murmurs / hx MI / HTN / HF / numb / tingle / cold extrem / slow wound healing
RESP	wheeze / SOB / cough / asthma / bronch / COPD
GI	abd pain / Δ in bowels / constipation / diarrhea / N V / hepatitis / gallstones / dysphagia / reflux / hemorrhoids / black, bloody stools
GU	burn / pain / nocturia / polyuria / hematuria / incontinence / infection / kid. stones
GENITAL	DC / sores / pain / masses / last pap _____ / sexually active Y N / dyspareunia / LMP _______ / contraception
MSK	redness / swelling / warmth / pain / +/- ROM / arthritis / musc cramps / fracture / sprains / joint replacement / stiffness: AM PM
SKIN	rash / pruritis / jaundice / bruising / hx skin ca / mole Δ / Δ in hair, nails / lesions / slow wound healing
BREASTS	lump / pain / dc / last mammo _______ / self exams YN
NEURO	HA / seizure / vertigo / memory Δ / gait Δ / speech / coord
PSYCH	depression / anxiety / Δ in sleep pattern / substance, ETOH abuse / suicidal ideation / homicidal ideation
ENDO	polydipsia, polyuria / heat, cold intolerance / Δ hair/nails/energy
HEM/LYMPH	anemia / bruising / hx transfusions / blood disorder / lymphadenopathy / axillary, groin tenderness
ALLX/IMMUN	season allx / food allx / med allx / immune disorder:

SOCIAL HX	# in household _______ / lives with SP/BF/GF/SO / children ___ / tobacco Y/N #pk / sexual activity Y/N / etoh, other substances Y/N / occupation:
FAM HX	ca / HTN / MI / CAD / stroke / hyperlipidemia / DM2 / Alzheimer's / depression / osteoporosis / other:

GENERAL	well appearing / well nourished / a&o x 3 / normal mood / normal affect
NEURO	intact / abnormal **DTR:** 1 2 3 4 5 location:
SKIN + NAILS	turgor / rash / bruising / lesions // texture, distribution of hair // nails: abnormal color / nail deformity
HEAD	normocephalic / atraumatic / visible mass / palpable mass / depression / scarring
EYES	acuity intact / conjunctiva clear / EOM intact / PERRLA / fundi: normal discs and vessels / icterus / exudate / hemorrhage
EARS	EACs clear / TM translucent, mobile / landmarks abnormal / hearing diminished
NOSE	lesions / mucosal inflammation / septum, turbinates abnormal / sinus tenderness
MOUTH	mucous membranes dry / lesions / poor dentition / caries / gingival inflammation
PHARYNX	mucosa inflammation / tonsillar hypertrophy / tonsillar exudate
NECK	supple / ROM WNL / lesion / bruit / adenopathy / thyroid enlarged, tender / mass
CARDIAC	regular rate, rhythm / S1, S2 / murmur / gallop / click / rub / PMI displacement
RESP	clear to auscultation in all fields / wheezes (insp) (exp) / rales / crackles
ABDOMEN	BSx4 / tender / organomegaly / mass / hernia
RECTAL	abnormal tone / hemorrhoids (int/ext) / palpable mass
BACK	abnormal curvature / tenderness / CVAT / Δ ROM
EXTREMITIES	amputation / deformity / edema / varicosities / + pulses
MSK	abnormal gait / asymmetry / crepitation / defect / tenderness / mass / effusion / Δ ROM / instability / atrophy / abnormal strength, tone in head, neck, spine, ribs, pelvis, UE, LE / pathologic reflexes
PSYCH	A&O x3 / +recent/remote memory / insight / affect
BREAST	nipple abnormality / mass / tenderness / axillary, clavicular adenopathy
GYN/GU	lesions / d/c / uterus, adnexa tenderness / CMT // circumcised / penile lesions / urethra normal location, no d/c / testes normal / + cremasteric reflex
FEET	+ pulses / monofilament + / nails abnormal / dry, broken skin / callus

LABS	CBC / CMP / lipids / TSH / microalbumin / A1C / UA, culture / PSA / iron studies / other:

DIAGNOSTICS	XR / MRI / CT / US / cardiac / other
REFERRALS	**F/U** ___ wk ___ mo

<table>
<tr><td colspan="2">

Patient ID#:

Reason for visit:
</td><td>

Date of visit:

Age: Gender:
</td></tr>
</table>

BP:	HT:
HR:	WT:
T:	BMI:
O2%:	PAIN:

NOTES . . . .

CONST	Δ appetite, energy, weight / fever / chills / sweats / fatigue
HEAD	trauma / mass / tenderness / rash / lesions
EYES	visionΔ / itch / d/c / tears / dry / cataracts / glaucoma / glasses, contacts
ENT	hearing Δ / pain / d/c / vertigo / ? infection // epistaxis / congestion // bleeding, swelling gums / pain / sore throat / voice Δ // neck pain / lumps / swelling / difficulty swallowing
CARDIAC	pain / pressure / dizzy / N / orthopnea / edema / palp / weak w exertion / hx murmurs / hx MI / HTN / HF / numb / tingle / cold extrem / slow wound healing
RESP	wheeze / SOB / cough / asthma / bronch / COPD
GI	abd pain / Δ in bowels / constipation / diarrhea / N V / hepatitis / gallstones / dysphagia / reflux / hemorrhoids / black, bloody stools
GU	burn / pain / nocturia / polyuria / hematuria / incontinence / infection / kid. stones
GENITAL	DC / sores / pain / masses / last pap _____ / sexually active Y N / dyspareunia / LMP _____ / contraception
MSK	redness / swelling / warmth / pain / +/- ROM / arthritis / musc cramps / fracture / sprains / joint replacement / stiffness: AM PM
SKIN	rash / pruritis / jaundice / bruising / hx skin ca / mole Δ / Δ in hair, nails / lesions / slow wound healing
BREASTS	lump / pain / dc / last mammo _____ / self exams YN
NEURO	HA / seizure / vertigo / memory Δ / gait Δ / speech / coord
PSYCH	depression / anxiety / Δ in sleep pattern / substance, ETOH abuse / suicidal ideation / homicidal ideation
ENDO	polydipsia, polyuria / heat, cold intolerance / Δ hair/nails/energy
HEM/LYMPH	anemia / bruising / hx transfusions / blood disorder / lymphadenopathy / axillary, groin tenderness
ALLX/IMMUN	season allx / food allx / med allx / immune disorder:

SOCIAL HX	# in household _____ / lives with SP/BF/GF/SO / children __ / tobacco Y/N #pk / sexual activity Y/N / etoh, other substances Y/N / occupation:
FAM HX	ca / HTN / MI / CAD / stroke / hyperlipidemia / DM2 / Alzheimer's / depression / osteoporosis / other:

GENERAL	well appearing / well nourished / a&o x 3 / normal mood / normal affect
NEURO	intact / abnormal **DTR:** 1 2 3 4 5 location:
SKIN + NAILS	turgor / rash / bruising / lesions // texture, distribution of hair // nails: abnormal color / nail deformity
HEAD	normocephalic / atraumatic / visible mass / palpable mass / depression / scarring
EYES	acuity intact / conjunctiva clear / EOM intact / PERRLA / fundi: normal discs and vessels / icterus / exudate / hemorrhage
EARS	EACs clear / TM translucent, mobile / landmarks abnormal / hearing diminished
NOSE	lesions / mucosal inflammation / septum, turbinates abnormal / sinus tenderness
MOUTH	mucous membranes dry / lesions / poor dentition / caries / gingival inflammation
PHARYNX	mucosa inflammation / tonsillar hypertrophy / tonsillar exudate
NECK	supple / ROM WNL / lesion / bruit / adenopathy / thyroid enlarged, tender / mass
CARDIAC	regular rate, rhythm / S1, S2 / murmur / gallop / click / rub / PMI displacement
RESP	clear to auscultation in all fields / wheezes (insp) (exp) / rales / crackles
ABDOMEN	BSx4 / tender / organomegaly / mass / hernia
RECTAL	abnormal tone / hemorrhoids (int/ext) / palpable mass
BACK	abnormal curvature / tenderness / CVAT / Δ ROM
EXTREMITIES	amputation / deformity / edema / varicosities / + pulses
MSK	abnormal gait / asymmetry / crepitation / defect / tenderness / mass / effusion / Δ ROM / instability / atrophy / abnormal strength, tone in head, neck, spine, ribs, pelvis, UE, LE / pathologic reflexes
PSYCH	A&O x3 / +recent/remote memory / insight / affect
BREAST	nipple abnormality / mass / tenderness / axillary, clavicular adenopathy
GYN/GU	lesions / d/c / uterus, adnexa tenderness / CMT // circumcised / penile lesions / urethra normal location, no d/c / testes normal / + cremasteric reflex
FEET	+ pulses / monofilament + / nails abnormal / dry, broken skin / callus

LABS	CBC / CMP / lipids / TSH / microalbumin / A1C / UA, culture / PSA / iron studies / other:

DIAGNOSTICS	XR / MRI / CT / US / cardiac / other
REFERRALS	**F/U** ___ wk ___ mo

<table>
<tr><td>Patient ID#:
Reason for visit:</td><td>Date of visit:
Age: Gender:</td></tr>
</table>

BP: HT:
HR: WT:
T: BMI:
O2%:   PAIN:

NOTES . . . .

CONST — Δ appetite, energy, weight / fever / chills / sweats / fatigue
HEAD — trauma / mass / tenderness / rash / lesions
EYES — visionΔ / itch / d/c / tears / dry / cataracts / glaucoma / glasses, contacts
ENT — hearing Δ / pain / d/c / vertigo / ? infection // epistaxis / congestion // bleeding, swelling gums / pain / sore throat / voice Δ // neck pain / lumps / swelling / difficulty swallowing

CARDIAC — pain / pressure / dizzy / N / orthopnea / edema / palp / weak w exertion / hx murmurs / hx MI / HTN / HF / numb / tingle / cold extrem / slow wound healing
RESP — wheeze / SOB / cough / asthma / bronch / COPD
GI — abd pain / Δ in bowels / constipation / diarrhea / N V / hepatitis / gallstones / dysphagia / reflux / hemorrhoids / black, bloody stools
GU — burn / pain / nocturia / polyuria / hematuria / incontinence / infection / kid. stones
GENITAL — DC / sores / pain / masses / last pap _____ / sexually active Y N / dyspareunia / LMP _______ / contraception
MSK — redness / swelling / warmth / pain / +/- ROM / arthritis / musc cramps / fracture / sprains / joint replacement / stiffness: AM PM
SKIN — rash / pruritis / jaundice / bruising / hx skin ca / mole Δ / Δ in hair, nails / lesions / slow wound healing
BREASTS — lump / pain / dc / last mammo _______ / self exams YN
NEURO — HA / seizure / vertigo / memory Δ / gait Δ / speech / coord
PSYCH — depression / anxiety / Δ in sleep pattern / substance, ETOH abuse / suicidal ideation / homicidal ideation
ENDO — polydipsia, polyuria / heat, cold intolerance / Δ hair/nails/energy
HEM/LYMPH — anemia / bruising / hx transfusions / blood disorder / lymphadenopathy / axillary, groin tenderness
ALLX/IMMUN — season allx / food allx / med allx / immune disorder:

SOCIAL HX — # in household _______ / lives with SP/BF/GF/SO / children __ / tobacco Y/N #pk / sexual activity Y/N / etoh, other substances Y/N / occupation:
FAM HX — ca / HTN / MI / CAD / stroke / hyperlipidemia / DM2 / Alzheimer's / depression / osteoporosis / other:

GENERAL — well appearing / well nourished / a&o x 3 / normal mood / normal affect
NEURO — intact / abnormal   **DTR:** 1 2 3 4 5 location:
SKIN + NAILS — turgor / rash / bruising / lesions // texture, distribution of hair // nails: abnormal color / nail deformity
HEAD — normocephalic / atraumatic / visible mass / palpable mass / depression / scarring
EYES — acuity intact / conjunctiva clear / EOM intact / PERRLA / fundi: normal discs and vessels / icterus / exudate / hemorrhage
EARS — EACs clear / TM translucent, mobile / landmarks abnormal / hearing diminished
NOSE — lesions / mucosal inflammation / septum, turbinates abnormal / sinus tenderness
MOUTH — mucous membranes dry / lesions / poor dentition / caries / gingival inflammation
PHARYNX — mucosa inflammation / tonsillar hypertrophy / tonsillar exudate
NECK — supple / ROM WNL / lesion / bruit / adenopathy / thyroid enlarged, tender / mass
CARDIAC — regular rate, rhythm / S1, S2 / murmur / gallop / click / rub / PMI displacement
RESP — clear to auscultation in all fields / wheezes (insp) (exp) / rales / crackles
ABDOMEN — BSx4 / tender / organomegaly / mass / hernia
RECTAL — abnormal tone / hemorrhoids (int/ext) / palpable mass
BACK — abnormal curvature / tenderness / CVAT / Δ ROM
EXTREMITIES — amputation / deformity / edema / varicosities / + pulses
MSK — abnormal gait / asymmetry / crepitation / defect / tenderness / mass / effusion / Δ ROM / instability / atrophy / abnormal strength, tone in head, neck, spine, ribs, pelvis, UE, LE / pathologic reflexes
PSYCH — A&O x3 / +recent/remote memory / insight / affect
BREAST — nipple abnormality / mass / tenderness / axillary, clavicular adenopathy
GYN/GU — lesions / d/c / uterus, adnexa tenderness / CMT // circumcised / penile lesions / urethra normal location, no d/c / testes normal / + cremasteric reflex
FEET — + pulses / monofilament + / nails abnormal / dry, broken skin / callus

LABS — CBC / CMP / lipids / TSH / microalbumin / A1C / UA, culture / PSA / iron studies / other:

DIAGNOSTICS — XR / MRI / CT / US / cardiac / other
REFERRALS —   **F/U** ___ wk ___ mo

<table>
<tr><td colspan="2">

Patient ID#:   **Date of visit:**

Reason for visit: **Age:**   **Gender:**

</td></tr>
</table>

BP:	**HT:**
HR:	**WT:**
T:	**BMI:**
O2%:	**PAIN:**

NOTES . . . .

CONST Δ appetite, energy, weight / fever / chills / sweats / fatigue

HEAD trauma / mass / tenderness / rash / lesions

EYES visionΔ / itch / d/c / tears / dry / cataracts / glaucoma / glasses, contacts

ENT hearing Δ / pain / d/c / vertigo / ? infection // epistaxis / congestion // bleeding, swelling gums / pain / sore throat / voice Δ // neck pain / lumps / swelling / difficulty swallowing

CARDIAC pain / pressure / dizzy / N / orthopnea / edema / palp / weak w exertion / hx murmurs / hx MI / HTN / HF / numb / tingle / cold extrem / slow wound healing

RESP wheeze / SOB / cough / asthma / bronch / COPD

GI abd pain / Δ in bowels / constipation / diarrhea / N V / hepatitis / gallstones / dysphagia / reflux / hemorrhoids / black, bloody stools

GU burn / pain / nocturia / polyuria / hematuria / incontinence / infection / kid. stones

GENITAL DC / sores / pain / masses / last pap ______ / sexually active Y N / dyspareunia / LMP ________ / contraception

MSK redness / swelling / warmth / pain / +/- ROM / arthritis / musc cramps / fracture / sprains / joint replacement / stiffness: AM PM

SKIN rash / pruritis / jaundice / bruising / hx skin ca / mole Δ / Δ in hair, nails / lesions / slow wound healing

BREASTS lump / pain / dc / last mammo ________ / self exams YN

NEURO HA / seizure / vertigo / memory Δ / gait Δ / speech / coord

PSYCH depression / anxiety / Δ in sleep pattern / substance, ETOH abuse / suicidal ideation / homicidal ideation

ENDO polydipsia, polyuria / heat, cold intolerance / Δ hair/nails/energy

HEM/LYMPH anemia / bruising / hx transfusions / blood disorder / lymphadenopathy / axillary, groin tenderness

ALLX/IMMUN season allx / food allx / med allx / immune disorder:

SOCIAL HX # in household ______ / lives with SP/BF/GF/SO / children __ / tobacco Y/N #pk / sexual activity Y/N / etoh, other substances Y/N / occupation:

FAM HX ca / HTN / MI / CAD / stroke / hyperlipidemia / DM2 / Alzheimer's / depression / osteoporosis / other:

GENERAL well appearing / well nourished / a&o x 3 / normal mood / normal affect

NEURO intact / abnormal   **DTR:** 1 2 3 4 5 location:

SKIN + NAILS turgor / rash / bruising / lesions // texture, distribution of hair // nails: abnormal color / nail deformity

HEAD normocephalic / atraumatic / visible mass / palpable mass / depression / scarring

EYES acuity intact / conjunctiva clear / EOM intact / PERRLA / fundi: normal discs and vessels / icterus / exudate / hemorrhage

EARS EACs clear / TM translucent, mobile / landmarks abnormal / hearing diminished

NOSE lesions / mucosal inflammation / septum, turbinates abnormal / sinus tenderness

MOUTH mucous membranes dry / lesions / poor dentition / caries / gingival inflammation

PHARYNX mucosa inflammation / tonsillar hypertrophy / tonsillar exudate

NECK supple / ROM WNL / lesion / bruit / adenopathy / thyroid enlarged, tender / mass

CARDIAC regular rate, rhythm / S1, S2 / murmur / gallop / click / rub / PMI displacement

RESP clear to auscultation in all fields / wheezes (insp) (exp) / rales / crackles

ABDOMEN BSx4 / tender / organomegaly / mass / hernia

RECTAL abnormal tone / hemorrhoids (int/ext) / palpable mass

BACK abnormal curvature / tenderness / CVAT / Δ ROM

EXTREMITIES amputation / deformity / edema / varicosities / + pulses

MSK abnormal gait / asymmetry / crepitation / defect / tenderness / mass / effusion / Δ ROM / instability / atrophy / abnormal strength, tone in head, neck, spine, ribs, pelvis, UE, LE / pathologic reflexes

PSYCH A&O x3 / +recent/remote memory / insight / affect

BREAST nipple abnormality / mass / tenderness / axillary, clavicular adenopathy

GYN/GU lesions / d/c / uterus, adnexa tenderness / CMT // circumcised / penile lesions / urethra normal location, no d/c / testes normal / + cremasteric reflex

FEET + pulses / monofilament + / nails abnormal / dry, broken skin / callus

---

LABS CBC / CMP / lipids / TSH / microalbumin / A1C / UA, culture / PSA / iron studies / other:

DIAGNOSTICS XR / MRI / CT / US / cardiac / other

REFERRALS   **F/U** ___ wk ___ mo

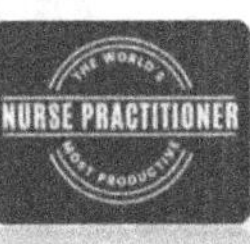

<table>
<tr><td colspan="2">

Patient ID#:　　　　　　　　**Date of visit:**
Reason for visit:　　　　　　**Age:**　**Gender:**

</td><td>

BP:　　　　　**HT:**
HR:　　　　　**WT:**
T:　　　　　　**BMI:**
O2%:　　　　**PAIN:**

</td></tr>
</table>

NOTES . . . .

CONST	Δ appetite, energy, weight / fever / chills / sweats / fatigue
HEAD	trauma / mass / tenderness / rash / lesions
EYES	visionΔ / itch / d/c / tears / dry / cataracts / glaucoma / glasses, contacts
ENT	hearing Δ / pain / d/c / vertigo / ? infection // epistaxis / congestion // bleeding, swelling gums / pain / sore throat / voice Δ // neck pain / lumps / swelling / difficulty swallowing
CARDIAC	pain / pressure / dizzy / N / orthopnea / edema / palp / weak w exertion / hx murmurs / hx MI / HTN / HF / numb / tingle / cold extrem / slow wound healing
RESP	wheeze / SOB / cough / asthma / bronch / COPD
GI	abd pain / Δ in bowels / constipation / diarrhea / N V / hepatitis / gallstones / dysphagia / reflux / hemorrhoids / black, bloody stools
GU	burn / pain / nocturia / polyuria / hematuria / incontinence / infection / kid. stones
GENITAL	DC / sores / pain / masses / last pap ______ / sexually active Y N / dyspareunia / LMP ______ / contraception
MSK	redness / swelling / warmth / pain / +/- ROM / arthritis / musc cramps / fracture / sprains / joint replacement / stiffness: AM PM
SKIN	rash / pruritis / jaundice / bruising / hx skin ca / mole Δ / Δ in hair, nails / lesions / slow wound healing
BREASTS	lump / pain / dc / last mammo ______ / self exams YN
NEURO	HA / seizure / vertigo / memory Δ / gait Δ / speech / coord
PSYCH	depression / anxiety / Δ in sleep pattern / substance, ETOH abuse / suicidal ideation / homicidal ideation
ENDO	polydipsia, polyuria / heat, cold intolerance / Δ hair/nails/energy
HEM/LYMPH	anemia / bruising / hx transfusions / blood disorder / lymphadenopathy / axillary, groin tenderness
ALLX/IMMUN	season allx / food allx / med allx / immune disorder:

SOCIAL HX	# in household ______ / lives with SP/BF/GF/SO / children __ / tobacco Y/N #pk / sexual activity Y/N / etoh, other substances Y/N / occupation:
FAM HX	ca / HTN / MI / CAD / stroke / hyperlipidemia / DM2 / Alzheimer's / depression / osteoporosis / other:

GENERAL	well appearing / well nourished / a&o x 3 / normal mood / normal affect
NEURO	intact / abnormal　　　　　　　**DTR:** 1 2 3 4 5 location:
SKIN + NAILS	turgor / rash / bruising / lesions // texture, distribution of hair // nails: abnormal color / nail deformity
HEAD	normocephalic / atraumatic / visible mass / palpable mass / depression / scarring
EYES	acuity intact / conjunctiva clear / EOM intact / PERRLA / fundi: normal discs and vessels / icterus / exudate / hemorrhage
EARS	EACs clear / TM translucent, mobile / landmarks abnormal / hearing diminished
NOSE	lesions / mucosal inflammation / septum, turbinates abnormal / sinus tenderness
MOUTH	mucous membranes dry / lesions / poor dentition / caries / gingival inflammation
PHARYNX	mucosa inflammation / tonsillar hypertrophy / tonsillar exudate
NECK	supple / ROM WNL / lesion / bruit / adenopathy / thyroid enlarged, tender / mass
CARDIAC	regular rate, rhythm / S1, S2 / murmur / gallop / click / rub / PMI displacement
RESP	clear to auscultation in all fields / wheezes (insp) (exp) / rales / crackles
ABDOMEN	BSx4 / tender / organomegaly / mass / hernia
RECTAL	abnormal tone / hemorrhoids (int/ext) / palpable mass
BACK	abnormal curvature / tenderness / CVAT / Δ ROM
EXTREMITIES	amputation / deformity / edema / varicosities / + pulses
MSK	abnormal gait / asymmetry / crepitation / defect / tenderness / mass / effusion / Δ ROM / instability / atrophy / abnormal strength, tone in head, neck, spine, ribs, pelvis, UE, LE / pathologic reflexes
PSYCH	A&O x3 / +recent/remote memory / insight / affect
BREAST	nipple abnormality / mass / tenderness / axillary, clavicular adenopathy
GYN/GU	lesions / d/c / uterus, adnexa tenderness / CMT // circumcised / penile lesions / urethra normal location, no d/c / testes normal / + cremasteric reflex
FEET	+ pulses / monofilament + / nails abnormal / dry, broken skin / callus

LABS	CBC / CMP / lipids / TSH / microalbumin / A1C / UA, culture / PSA / iron studies / other:

DIAGNOSTICS	XR / MRI / CT / US / cardiac / other
REFERRALS	**F/U** ___ wk ___ mo

<table>
<tr><td>Patient ID#:</td><td>Date of visit:</td></tr>
<tr><td>Reason for visit:</td><td>Age: Gender:</td></tr>
</table>

BP:	HT:
HR:	WT:
T:	BMI:
O2%:	PAIN:

NOTES . . . .

CONST	Δ appetite, energy, weight / fever / chills / sweats / fatigue
HEAD	trauma / mass / tenderness / rash / lesions
EYES	visionΔ / itch / d/c / tears / dry / cataracts / glaucoma / glasses, contacts
ENT	hearing Δ / pain / d/c / vertigo / ? infection // epistaxis / congestion // bleeding, swelling gums / pain / sore throat / voice Δ // neck pain / lumps / swelling / difficulty swallowing
CARDIAC	pain / pressure / dizzy / N / orthopnea / edema / palp / weak w exertion / hx murmurs / hx MI / HTN / HF / numb / tingle / cold extrem / slow wound healing
RESP	wheeze / SOB / cough / asthma / bronch / COPD
GI	abd pain / Δ in bowels / constipation / diarrhea / N V / hepatitis / gallstones / dysphagia / reflux / hemorrhoids / black, bloody stools
GU	burn / pain / nocturia / polyuria / hematuria / incontinence / infection / kid. stones
GENITAL	DC / sores / pain / masses / last pap _____ / sexually active Y N / dyspareunia / LMP _____ / contraception
MSK	redness / swelling / warmth / pain / +/- ROM / arthritis / musc cramps / fracture / sprains / joint replacement / stiffness: AM PM
SKIN	rash / pruritis / jaundice / bruising / hx skin ca / mole Δ / Δ in hair, nails / lesions / slow wound healing
BREASTS	lump / pain / dc / last mammo _____ / self exams YN
NEURO	HA / seizure / vertigo / memory Δ / gait Δ / speech / coord
PSYCH	depression / anxiety / Δ in sleep pattern / substance, ETOH abuse / suicidal ideation / homicidal ideation
ENDO	polydipsia, polyuria / heat, cold intolerance / Δ hair/nails/energy
HEM/LYMPH	anemia / bruising / hx transfusions / blood disorder / lymphadenopathy / axillary, groin tenderness
ALLX/IMMUN	season allx / food allx / med allx / immune disorder:
SOCIAL HX	# in household _____ / lives with SP/BF/GF/SO / children __ / tobacco Y/N #pk / sexual activity Y/N / etoh, other substances Y/N / occupation:
FAM HX	ca / HTN / MI / CAD / stroke / hyperlipidemia / DM2 / Alzheimer's / depression / osteoporosis / other:
GENERAL	well appearing / well nourished / a&o x 3 / normal mood / normal affect
NEURO	intact / abnormal **DTR:** 1 2 3 4 5 location:
SKIN + NAILS	turgor / rash / bruising / lesions // texture, distribution of hair // nails: abnormal color / nail deformity
HEAD	normocephalic / atraumatic / visible mass / palpable mass / depression / scarring
EYES	acuity intact / conjunctiva clear / EOM intact / PERRLA / fundi: normal discs and vessels / icterus / exudate / hemorrhage
EARS	EACs clear / TM translucent, mobile / landmarks abnormal / hearing diminished
NOSE	lesions / mucosal inflammation / septum, turbinates abnormal / sinus tenderness
MOUTH	mucous membranes dry / lesions / poor dentition / caries / gingival inflammation
PHARYNX	mucosa inflammation / tonsillar hypertrophy / tonsillar exudate
NECK	supple / ROM WNL / lesion / bruit / adenopathy / thyroid enlarged, tender / mass
CARDIAC	regular rate, rhythm / S1, S2 / murmur / gallop / click / rub / PMI displacement
RESP	clear to auscultation in all fields / wheezes (insp) (exp) / rales / crackles
ABDOMEN	BSx4 / tender / organomegaly / mass / hernia
RECTAL	abnormal tone / hemorrhoids (int/ext) / palpable mass
BACK	abnormal curvature / tenderness / CVAT / Δ ROM
EXTREMITIES	amputation / deformity / edema / varicosities / + pulses
MSK	abnormal gait / asymmetry / crepitation / defect / tenderness / mass / effusion / Δ ROM / instability / atrophy / abnormal strength, tone in head, neck, spine, ribs, pelvis, UE, LE / pathologic reflexes
PSYCH	A&O x3 / +recent/remote memory / insight / affect
BREAST	nipple abnormality / mass / tenderness / axillary, clavicular adenopathy
GYN/GU	lesions / d/c / uterus, adnexa tenderness / CMT // circumcised / penile lesions / urethra normal location, no d/c / testes normal / + cremasteric reflex
FEET	+ pulses / monofilament + / nails abnormal / dry, broken skin / callus
LABS	CBC / CMP / lipids / TSH / microalbumin / A1C / UA, culture / PSA / iron studies / other:
DIAGNOSTICS	XR / MRI / CT / US / cardiac / other
REFERRALS	**F/U** ___ wk ___ mo

<table>
<tr><td>

Patient ID#:

Reason for visit:

</td><td>

Date of visit:

Age: Gender:

</td></tr>
</table>

BP: **HT:**
HR: **WT:**
T: **BMI:**
O2%:   **PAIN:**

NOTES . . . .

CONST Δ appetite, energy, weight / fever / chills / sweats / fatigue
HEAD trauma / mass / tenderness / rash / lesions
EYES visionΔ / itch / d/c / tears / dry / cataracts / glaucoma / glasses, contacts
ENT hearing Δ / pain / d/c / vertigo / ? infection // epistaxis / congestion // bleeding, swelling gums / pain / sore throat / voice Δ // neck pain / lumps / swelling / difficulty swallowing
CARDIAC pain / pressure / dizzy / N / orthopnea / edema / palp / weak w exertion / hx murmurs / hx MI / HTN / HF / numb / tingle / cold extrem / slow wound healing
RESP wheeze / SOB / cough / asthma / bronch / COPD
GI abd pain / Δ in bowels / constipation / diarrhea / N V / hepatitis / gallstones / dysphagia / reflux / hemorrhoids / black, bloody stools
GU burn / pain / nocturia / polyuria / hematuria / incontinence / infection / kid. stones
GENITAL DC / sores / pain / masses / last pap _______ / sexually active Y N / dyspareunia / LMP _________ / contraception
MSK redness / swelling / warmth / pain / +/- ROM / arthritis / musc cramps / fracture / sprains / joint replacement / stiffness: AM PM
SKIN rash / pruritis / jaundice / bruising / hx skin ca / mole Δ / Δ in hair, nails / lesions / slow wound healing
BREASTS lump / pain / dc / last mammo _______ / self exams YN
NEURO HA / seizure / vertigo / memory Δ / gait Δ / speech / coord
PSYCH depression / anxiety / Δ in sleep pattern / substance, ETOH abuse / suicidal ideation / homicidal ideation
ENDO polydipsia, polyuria / heat, cold intolerance / Δ hair/nails/energy
HEM/LYMPH anemia / bruising / hx transfusions / blood disorder / lymphadenopathy / axillary, groin tenderness
ALLX/IMMUN season allx / food allx / med allx / immune disorder:

SOCIAL HX # in household _______ / lives with SP/BF/GF/SO / children __ / tobacco Y/N #pk / sexual activity Y/N / etoh, other substances Y/N / occupation:
FAM HX ca / HTN / MI / CAD / stroke / hyperlipidemia / DM2 / Alzheimer's / depression / osteoporosis / other:

GENERAL well appearing / well nourished / a&o x 3 / normal mood / normal affect
NEURO intact / abnormal   **DTR:** 1 2 3 4 5 location:
SKIN + NAILS turgor / rash / bruising / lesions // texture, distribution of hair // nails: abnormal color / nail deformity
HEAD normocephalic / atraumatic / visible mass / palpable mass / depression / scarring
EYES acuity intact / conjunctiva clear / EOM intact / PERRLA / fundi: normal discs and vessels / icterus / exudate / hemorrhage
EARS EACs clear / TM translucent, mobile / landmarks abnormal / hearing diminished
NOSE lesions / mucosal inflammation / septum, turbinates abnormal / sinus tenderness
MOUTH mucous membranes dry / lesions / poor dentition / caries / gingival inflammation
PHARYNX mucosa inflammation / tonsillar hypertrophy / tonsillar exudate
NECK supple / ROM WNL / lesion / bruit / adenopathy / thyroid enlarged, tender / mass
CARDIAC regular rate, rhythm / S1, S2 / murmur / gallop / click / rub / PMI displacement
RESP clear to auscultation in all fields / wheezes (insp) (exp) / rales / crackles
ABDOMEN BSx4 / tender / organomegaly / mass / hernia
RECTAL abnormal tone / hemorrhoids (int/ext) / palpable mass
BACK abnormal curvature / tenderness / CVAT / Δ ROM
EXTREMITIES amputation / deformity / edema / varicosities / + pulses
MSK abnormal gait / asymmetry / crepitation / defect / tenderness / mass / effusion / Δ ROM / instability / atrophy / abnormal strength, tone in head, neck, spine, ribs, pelvis, UE, LE / pathologic reflexes
PSYCH A&O x3 / +recent/remote memory / insight / affect
BREAST nipple abnormality / mass / tenderness / axillary, clavicular adenopathy
GYN/GU lesions / d/c / uterus, adnexa tenderness / CMT // circumcised / penile lesions / urethra normal location, no d/c / testes normal / + cremasteric reflex
FEET + pulses / monofilament + / nails abnormal / dry, broken skin / callus

LABS CBC / CMP / lipids / TSH / microalbumin / A1C / UA, culture / PSA / iron studies / other:

DIAGNOSTICS XR / MRI / CT / US / cardiac / other
REFERRALS   **F/U** ___ wk ___ mo

<table>
<tr><td>Patient ID#:</td><td>Date of visit:</td></tr>
<tr><td>Reason for visit:</td><td>Age: Gender:</td></tr>
</table>

BP: HT:
HR: WT:
T: BMI:
O2%:   PAIN:

NOTES . . . .

CONST Δ appetite, energy, weight / fever / chills / sweats / fatigue
HEAD trauma / mass / tenderness / rash / lesions
EYES visionΔ / itch / d/c / tears / dry / cataracts / glaucoma / glasses, contacts
ENT hearing Δ / pain / d/c / vertigo / ? infection // epistaxis / congestion // bleeding, swelling gums / pain / sore throat / voice Δ // neck pain / lumps / swelling / difficulty swallowing

CARDIAC pain / pressure / dizzy / N / orthopnea / edema / palp / weak w exertion / hx murmurs / hx MI / HTN / HF / numb / tingle / cold extrem / slow wound healing

RESP wheeze / SOB / cough / asthma / bronch / COPD
GI abd pain / Δ in bowels / constipation / diarrhea / N V / hepatitis / gallstones / dysphagia / reflux / hemorrhoids / black, bloody stools

GU burn / pain / nocturia / polyuria / hematuria / incontinence / infection / kid. stones
GENITAL DC / sores / pain / masses / last pap _______ / sexually active Y N / dyspareunia / LMP _______ / contraception

MSK redness / swelling / warmth / pain / +/- ROM / arthritis / musc cramps / fracture / sprains / joint replacement / stiffness: AM PM

SKIN rash / pruritis / jaundice / bruising / hx skin ca / mole Δ / Δ in hair, nails / lesions / slow wound healing

BREASTS lump / pain / dc / last mammo _______ / self exams YN
NEURO HA / seizure / vertigo / memory Δ / gait Δ / speech / coord
PSYCH depression / anxiety / Δ in sleep pattern / substance, ETOH abuse / suicidal ideation / homicidal ideation

ENDO polydipsia, polyuria / heat, cold intolerance / Δ hair/nails/energy
HEM/LYMPH anemia / bruising / hx transfusions / blood disorder / lymphadenopathy / axillary, groin tenderness

ALLX/IMMUN season allx / food allx / med allx / immune disorder:

SOCIAL HX # in household _______ / lives with SP/BF/GF/SO / children __ / tobacco Y/N #pk / sexual activity Y/N / etoh, other substances Y/N / occupation:

FAM HX ca / HTN / MI / CAD / stroke / hyperlipidemia / DM2 / Alzheimer's / depression / osteoporosis / other:

GENERAL well appearing / well nourished / a&o x 3 / normal mood / normal affect
NEURO intact / abnormal   **DTR:** 1 2 3 4 5 location:
SKIN + NAILS turgor / rash / bruising / lesions // texture, distribution of hair // nails: abnormal color / nail deformity

HEAD normocephalic / atraumatic / visible mass / palpable mass / depression / scarring
EYES acuity intact / conjunctiva clear / EOM intact / PERRLA / fundi: normal discs and vessels / icterus / exudate / hemorrhage

EARS EACs clear / TM translucent, mobile / landmarks abnormal / hearing diminished
NOSE lesions / mucosal inflammation / septum, turbinates abnormal / sinus tenderness
MOUTH mucous membranes dry / lesions / poor dentition / caries / gingival inflammation
PHARYNX mucosa inflammation / tonsillar hypertrophy / tonsillar exudate
NECK supple / ROM WNL / lesion / bruit / adenopathy / thyroid enlarged, tender / mass
CARDIAC regular rate, rhythm / S1, S2 / murmur / gallop / click / rub / PMI displacement
RESP clear to auscultation in all fields / wheezes (insp) (exp) / rales / crackles
ABDOMEN BSx4 / tender / organomegaly / mass / hernia
RECTAL abnormal tone / hemorrhoids (int/ext) / palpable mass
BACK abnormal curvature / tenderness / CVAT / Δ ROM
EXTREMITIES amputation / deformity / edema / varicosities / + pulses
MSK abnormal gait / asymmetry / crepitation / defect / tenderness / mass / effusion / Δ ROM / instability / atrophy / abnormal strength, tone in head, neck, spine, ribs, pelvis, UE, LE / pathologic reflexes

PSYCH A&O x3 / +recent/remote memory / insight / affect
BREAST nipple abnormality / mass / tenderness / axillary, clavicular adenopathy
GYN/GU lesions / d/c / uterus, adnexa tenderness / CMT // circumcised / penile lesions / urethra normal location, no d/c / testes normal / + cremasteric reflex
FEET + pulses / monofilament + / nails abnormal / dry, broken skin / callus

---

LABS CBC / CMP / lipids / TSH / microalbumin / A1C / UA, culture / PSA / iron studies / other:

DIAGNOSTICS XR / MRI / CT / US / cardiac / other
REFERRALS   **F/U** ___ wk ___ mo

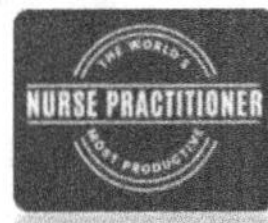

<table>
<tr><td>Patient ID#:</td><td>Date of visit:</td></tr>
<tr><td>Reason for visit:</td><td>Age: Gender:</td></tr>
</table>

BP:	HT:
HR:	WT:
T:	BMI:
O2%:	PAIN:

NOTES . . . .

CONST	Δ appetite, energy, weight / fever / chills / sweats / fatigue
HEAD	trauma / mass / tenderness / rash / lesions
EYES	visionΔ / itch / d/c / tears / dry / cataracts / glaucoma / glasses, contacts
ENT	hearing Δ / pain / d/c / vertigo / ? infection // epistaxis / congestion // bleeding, swelling gums / pain / sore throat / voice Δ // neck pain / lumps / swelling / difficulty swallowing
CARDIAC	pain / pressure / dizzy / N / orthopnea / edema / palp / weak w exertion / hx murmurs / hx MI / HTN / HF / numb / tingle / cold extrem / slow wound healing
RESP	wheeze / SOB / cough / asthma / bronch / COPD
GI	abd pain / Δ in bowels / constipation / diarrhea / N V / hepatitis / gallstones / dysphagia / reflux / hemorrhoids / black, bloody stools
GU	burn / pain / nocturia / polyuria / hematuria / incontinence / infection / kid. stones
GENITAL	DC / sores / pain / masses / last pap _____ / sexually active Y N / dyspareunia / LMP / contraception
MSK	redness / swelling / warmth / pain / +/- ROM / arthritis / musc cramps / fracture / sprains / joint replacement / stiffness: AM PM
SKIN	rash / pruritis / jaundice / bruising / hx skin ca / mole Δ / Δ in hair, nails / lesions / slow wound healing
BREASTS	lump / pain / dc / last mammo / self exams YN
NEURO	HA / seizure / vertigo / memory Δ / gait Δ / speech / coord
PSYCH	depression / anxiety / Δ in sleep pattern / substance, ETOH abuse / suicidal ideation / homicidal ideation
ENDO	polydipsia, polyuria / heat, cold intolerance / Δ hair/nails/energy
HEM/LYMPH	anemia / bruising / hx transfusions / blood disorder / lymphadenopathy / axillary, groin tenderness
ALLX/IMMUN	season allx / food allx / med allx / immune disorder:

SOCIAL HX	# in household _____ / lives with SP/BF/GF/SO / children __ / tobacco Y/N #pk / sexual activity Y/N / etoh, other substances Y/N / occupation:
FAM HX	ca / HTN / MI / CAD / stroke / hyperlipidemia / DM2 / Alzheimer's / depression / osteoporosis / other:

GENERAL	well appearing / well nourished / a&o x 3 / normal mood / normal affect
NEURO	intact / abnormal **DTR:** 1 2 3 4 5 location:
SKIN + NAILS	turgor / rash / bruising / lesions // texture, distribution of hair // nails: abnormal color / nail deformity
HEAD	normocephalic / atraumatic / visible mass / palpable mass / depression / scarring
EYES	acuity intact / conjunctiva clear / EOM intact / PERRLA / fundi: normal discs and vessels / icterus / exudate / hemorrhage
EARS	EACs clear / TM translucent, mobile / landmarks abnormal / hearing diminished
NOSE	lesions / mucosal inflammation / septum, turbinates abnormal / sinus tenderness
MOUTH	mucous membranes dry / lesions / poor dentition / caries / gingival inflammation
PHARYNX	mucosa inflammation / tonsillar hypertrophy / tonsillar exudate
NECK	supple / ROM WNL / lesion / bruit / adenopathy / thyroid enlarged, tender / mass
CARDIAC	regular rate, rhythm / S1, S2 / murmur / gallop / click / rub / PMI displacement
RESP	clear to auscultation in all fields / wheezes (insp) (exp) / rales / crackles
ABDOMEN	BSx4 / tender / organomegaly / mass / hernia
RECTAL	abnormal tone / hemorrhoids (int/ext) / palpable mass
BACK	abnormal curvature / tenderness / CVAT / Δ ROM
EXTREMITIES	amputation / deformity / edema / varicosities / + pulses
MSK	abnormal gait / asymmetry / crepitation / defect / tenderness / mass / effusion / Δ ROM / instability / atrophy / abnormal strength, tone in head, neck, spine, ribs, pelvis, UE, LE / pathologic reflexes
PSYCH	A&O x3 / +recent/remote memory / insight / affect
BREAST	nipple abnormality / mass / tenderness / axillary, clavicular adenopathy
GYN/GU	lesions / d/c / uterus, adnexa tenderness / CMT // circumcised / penile lesions / urethra normal location, no d/c / testes normal / + cremasteric reflex
FEET	+ pulses / monofilament + / nails abnormal / dry, broken skin / callus

LABS	CBC / CMP / lipids / TSH / microalbumin / A1C / UA, culture / PSA / iron studies / other:

DIAGNOSTICS	XR / MRI / CT / US / cardiac / other
REFERRALS	**F/U** ___ wk ___ mo

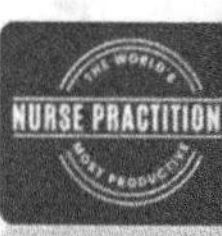

<table>
<tr><td>

Patient ID#:

Reason for visit:

</td><td>

Date of visit:

Age: **Gender:**

</td></tr>
</table>

BP:	HT:
HR:	WT:
T:	BMI:
O2%:	PAIN:

NOTES . . . .

CONST	Δ appetite, energy, weight / fever / chills / sweats / fatigue
HEAD	trauma / mass / tenderness / rash / lesions
EYES	visionΔ / itch / d/c / tears / dry / cataracts / glaucoma / glasses, contacts
ENT	hearing Δ / pain / d/c / vertigo / ? infection // epistaxis / congestion // bleeding, swelling gums / pain / sore throat / voice Δ // neck pain / lumps / swelling / difficulty swallowing
CARDIAC	pain / pressure / dizzy / N / orthopnea / edema / palp / weak w exertion / hx murmurs / hx MI / HTN / HF / numb / tingle / cold extrem / slow wound healing
RESP	wheeze / SOB / cough / asthma / bronch / COPD
GI	abd pain / Δ in bowels / constipation / diarrhea / N V / hepatitis / gallstones / dysphagia / reflux / hemorrhoids / black, bloody stools
GU	burn / pain / nocturia / polyuria / hematuria / incontinence / infection / kid. stones
GENITAL	DC / sores / pain / masses / last pap _____ / sexually active Y N / dyspareunia / LMP _______ / contraception
MSK	redness / swelling / warmth / pain / +/- ROM / arthritis / musc cramps / fracture / sprains / joint replacement / stiffness: AM PM
SKIN	rash / pruritis / jaundice / bruising / hx skin ca / mole Δ / Δ in hair, nails / lesions / slow wound healing
BREASTS	lump / pain / dc / last mammo _______ / self exams YN
NEURO	HA / seizure / vertigo / memory Δ / gait Δ / speech / coord
PSYCH	depression / anxiety / Δ in sleep pattern / substance, ETOH abuse / suicidal ideation / homicidal ideation
ENDO	polydipsia, polyuria / heat, cold intolerance / Δ hair/nails/energy
HEM/LYMPH	anemia / bruising / hx transfusions / blood disorder / lymphadenopathy / axillary, groin tenderness
ALLX/IMMUN	season allx / food allx / med allx / immune disorder:

SOCIAL HX	# in household _______ / lives with SP/BF/GF/SO / children __ / tobacco Y/N #pk / sexual activity Y/N / etoh, other substances Y/N / occupation:
FAM HX	ca / HTN / MI / CAD / stroke / hyperlipidemia / DM2 / Alzheimer's / depression / osteoporosis / other:

GENERAL	well appearing / well nourished / a&o x 3 / normal mood / normal affect
NEURO	intact / abnormal **DTR:** 1 2 3 4 5 location:
SKIN + NAILS	turgor / rash / bruising / lesions // texture, distribution of hair // nails: abnormal color / nail deformity
HEAD	normocephalic / atraumatic / visible mass / palpable mass / depression / scarring
EYES	acuity intact / conjunctiva clear / EOM intact / PERRLA / fundi: normal discs and vessels / icterus / exudate / hemorrhage
EARS	EACs clear / TM translucent, mobile / landmarks abnormal / hearing diminished
NOSE	lesions / mucosal inflammation / septum, turbinates abnormal / sinus tenderness
MOUTH	mucous membranes dry / lesions / poor dentition / caries / gingival inflammation
PHARYNX	mucosa inflammation / tonsillar hypertrophy / tonsillar exudate
NECK	supple / ROM WNL / lesion / bruit / adenopathy / thyroid enlarged, tender / mass
CARDIAC	regular rate, rhythm / S1, S2 / murmur / gallop / click / rub / PMI displacement
RESP	clear to auscultation in all fields / wheezes (insp) (exp) / rales / crackles
ABDOMEN	BSx4 / tender / organomegaly / mass / hernia
RECTAL	abnormal tone / hemorrhoids (int/ext) / palpable mass
BACK	abnormal curvature / tenderness / CVAT / Δ ROM
EXTREMITIES	amputation / deformity / edema / varicosities / + pulses
MSK	abnormal gait / asymmetry / crepitation / defect / tenderness / mass / effusion / Δ ROM / instability / atrophy / abnormal strength, tone in head, neck, spine, ribs, pelvis, UE, LE / pathologic reflexes
PSYCH	A&O x3 / +recent/remote memory / insight / affect
BREAST	nipple abnormality / mass / tenderness / axillary, clavicular adenopathy
GYN/GU	lesions / d/c / uterus, adnexa tenderness / CMT // circumcised / penile lesions / urethra normal location, no d/c / testes normal / + cremasteric reflex
FEET	+ pulses / monofilament + / nails abnormal / dry, broken skin / callus

LABS	CBC / CMP / lipids / TSH / microalbumin / A1C / UA, culture / PSA / iron studies / other:

DIAGNOSTICS	XR / MRI / CT / US / cardiac / other
REFERRALS	**F/U** ___ wk ___ mo

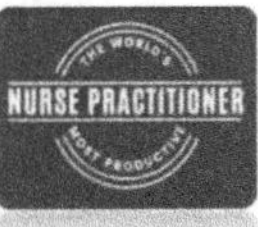

<table>
<tr><td>

Patient ID#:	Date of visit:
Reason for visit:	Age: Gender:

</td><td>

BP:	HT:
HR:	WT:
T:	BMI:
O2%:	PAIN:

NOTES . . . .

</td></tr>
</table>

CONST   Δ appetite, energy, weight / fever / chills / sweats / fatigue
HEAD   trauma / mass / tenderness / rash / lesions
EYES   visionΔ / itch / d/c / tears / dry / cataracts / glaucoma / glasses, contacts
ENT   hearing Δ / pain / d/c / vertigo / ? infection // epistaxis / congestion // bleeding, swelling gums / pain / sore throat / voice Δ // neck pain / lumps / swelling / difficulty swallowing

CARDIAC   pain / pressure / dizzy / N / orthopnea / edema / palp / weak w exertion / hx murmurs / hx MI / HTN / HF / numb / tingle / cold extrem / slow wound healing

RESP   wheeze / SOB / cough / asthma / bronch / COPD
GI   abd pain / Δ in bowels / constipation / diarrhea / N V / hepatitis / gallstones / dysphagia / reflux / hemorrhoids / black, bloody stools

GU   burn / pain / nocturia / polyuria / hematuria / incontinence / infection / kid. stones
GENITAL   DC / sores / pain / masses / last pap _______ / sexually active Y N / dyspareunia / LMP _______ / contraception

MSK   redness / swelling / warmth / pain / +/- ROM / arthritis / musc cramps / fracture / sprains / joint replacement / stiffness: AM PM

SKIN   rash / pruritis / jaundice / bruising / hx skin ca / mole Δ / Δ in hair, nails / lesions / slow wound healing

BREASTS   lump / pain / dc / last mammo _______ / self exams YN
NEURO   HA / seizure / vertigo / memory Δ / gait Δ / speech / coord
PSYCH   depression / anxiety / Δ in sleep pattern / substance, ETOH abuse / suicidal ideation / homicidal ideation

ENDO   polydipsia, polyuria / heat, cold intolerance / Δ hair/nails/energy
HEM/LYMPH   anemia / bruising / hx transfusions / blood disorder / lymphadenopathy / axillary, groin tenderness

ALLX/IMMUN   season allx / food allx / med allx / immune disorder:

SOCIAL HX   # in household _______ / lives with SP/BF/GF/SO / children ___ / tobacco Y/N #pk / sexual activity Y/N / etoh, other substances Y/N / occupation:
FAM HX   ca / HTN / MI / CAD / stroke / hyperlipidemia / DM2 / Alzheimer's / depression / osteoporosis / other:

GENERAL   well appearing / well nourished / a&o x 3 / normal mood / normal affect
NEURO   intact / abnormal   **DTR:** 1 2 3 4 5 location:
SKIN + NAILS   turgor / rash / bruising / lesions // texture, distribution of hair // nails: abnormal color / nail deformity

HEAD   normocephalic / atraumatic / visible mass / palpable mass / depression / scarring
EYES   acuity intact / conjunctiva clear / EOM intact / PERRLA / fundi: normal discs and vessels / icterus / exudate / hemorrhage

EARS   EACs clear / TM translucent, mobile / landmarks abnormal / hearing diminished
NOSE   lesions / mucosal inflammation / septum, turbinates abnormal / sinus tenderness
MOUTH   mucous membranes dry / lesions / poor dentition / caries / gingival inflammation
PHARYNX   mucosa inflammation / tonsillar hypertrophy / tonsillar exudate
NECK   supple / ROM WNL / lesion / bruit / adenopathy / thyroid enlarged, tender / mass
CARDIAC   regular rate, rhythm / S1, S2 / murmur / gallop / click / rub / PMI displacement
RESP   clear to auscultation in all fields / wheezes (insp) (exp) / rales / crackles
ABDOMEN   BSx4 / tender / organomegaly / mass / hernia
RECTAL   abnormal tone / hemorrhoids (int/ext) / palpable mass
BACK   abnormal curvature / tenderness / CVAT / Δ ROM
EXTREMITIES   amputation / deformity / edema / varicosities / + pulses
MSK   abnormal gait / asymmetry / crepitation / defect / tenderness / mass / effusion / Δ ROM / instability / atrophy / abnormal strength, tone in head, neck, spine, ribs, pelvis, UE, LE / pathologic reflexes

PSYCH   A&O x3 / +recent/remote memory / insight / affect
BREAST   nipple abnormality / mass / tenderness / axillary, clavicular adenopathy
GYN/GU   lesions / d/c / uterus, adnexa tenderness / CMT // circumcised / penile lesions / urethra normal location, no d/c / testes normal / + cremasteric reflex
FEET   + pulses / monofilament + / nails abnormal / dry, broken skin / callus

---

LABS   CBC / CMP / lipids / TSH / microalbumin / A1C / UA, culture / PSA / iron studies / other:

DIAGNOSTICS   XR / MRI / CT / US / cardiac / other
REFERRALS   **F/U** ___ wk ___ mo

<table>
<tr><td colspan="2">
Patient ID#:
Reason for visit:
</td><td>
Date of visit:
Age: Gender:
</td></tr>
</table>

BP:	**HT:**	
HR:	**WT:**	
T:	**BMI:**	
O2%:	**PAIN:**	

NOTES . . . .

CONST Δ appetite, energy, weight / fever / chills / sweats / fatigue
HEAD trauma / mass / tenderness / rash / lesions
EYES visionΔ / itch / d/c / tears / dry / cataracts / glaucoma / glasses, contacts
ENT hearing Δ / pain / d/c / vertigo / ? infection // epistaxis / congestion // bleeding, swelling gums / pain / sore throat / voice Δ // neck pain / lumps / swelling / difficulty swallowing

CARDIAC pain / pressure / dizzy / N / orthopnea / edema / palp / weak w exertion / hx murmurs / hx MI / HTN / HF / numb / tingle / cold extrem / slow wound healing

RESP wheeze / SOB / cough / asthma / bronch / COPD
GI abd pain / Δ in bowels / constipation / diarrhea / N V / hepatitis / gallstones / dysphagia / reflux / hemorrhoids / black, bloody stools

GU burn / pain / nocturia / polyuria / hematuria / incontinence / infection / kid. stones
GENITAL DC / sores / pain / masses / last pap _______ / sexually active Y N / dyspareunia / LMP _________ / contraception

MSK redness / swelling / warmth / pain / +/- ROM / arthritis / musc cramps / fracture / sprains / joint replacement / stiffness: AM PM

SKIN rash / pruritis / jaundice / bruising / hx skin ca / mole Δ / Δ in hair, nails / lesions / slow wound healing

BREASTS lump / pain / dc / last mammo _________ / self exams YN
NEURO HA / seizure / vertigo / memory Δ / gait Δ / speech / coord
PSYCH depression / anxiety / Δ in sleep pattern / substance, ETOH abuse / suicidal ideation / homicidal ideation

ENDO polydipsia, polyuria / heat, cold intolerance / Δ hair/nails/energy
HEM/LYMPH anemia / bruising / hx transfusions / blood disorder / lymphadenopathy / axillary, groin tenderness

ALLX/IMMUN season allx / food allx / med allx / immune disorder:

SOCIAL HX # in household _______ / lives with SP/BF/GF/SO / children __ / tobacco Y/N #pk / sexual activity Y/N / etoh, other substances Y/N / occupation:

FAM HX ca / HTN / MI / CAD / stroke / hyperlipidemia / DM2 / Alzheimer's / depression / osteoporosis / other:

GENERAL well appearing / well nourished / a&o x 3 / normal mood / normal affect
NEURO intact / abnormal **DTR:** 1 2 3 4 5 location:
SKIN + NAILS turgor / rash / bruising / lesions // texture, distribution of hair // nails: abnormal color / nail deformity

HEAD normocephalic / atraumatic / visible mass / palpable mass / depression / scarring
EYES acuity intact / conjunctiva clear / EOM intact / PERRLA / fundi: normal discs and vessels / icterus / exudate / hemorrhage

EARS EACs clear / TM translucent, mobile / landmarks abnormal / hearing diminished
NOSE lesions / mucosal inflammation / septum, turbinates abnormal / sinus tenderness
MOUTH mucous membranes dry / lesions / poor dentition / caries / gingival inflammation
PHARYNX mucosa inflammation / tonsillar hypertrophy / tonsillar exudate
NECK supple / ROM WNL / lesion / bruit / adenopathy / thyroid enlarged, tender / mass
CARDIAC regular rate, rhythm / S1, S2 / murmur / gallop / click / rub / PMI displacement
RESP clear to auscultation in all fields / wheezes (insp) (exp) / rales / crackles
ABDOMEN BSx4 / tender / organomegaly / mass / hernia
RECTAL abnormal tone / hemorrhoids (int/ext) / palpable mass
BACK abnormal curvature / tenderness / CVAT / Δ ROM
EXTREMITIES amputation / deformity / edema / varicosities / + pulses
MSK abnormal gait / asymmetry / crepitation / defect / tenderness / mass / effusion / Δ ROM / instability / atrophy / abnormal strength, tone in head, neck, spine, ribs, pelvis, UE, LE / pathologic reflexes

PSYCH A&O x3 / +recent/remote memory / insight / affect
BREAST nipple abnormality / mass / tenderness / axillary, clavicular adenopathy
GYN/GU lesions / d/c / uterus, adnexa tenderness / CMT // circumcised / penile lesions / urethra normal location, no d/c / testes normal / + cremasteric reflex
FEET + pulses / monofilament + / nails abnormal / dry, broken skin / callus

---

LABS CBC / CMP / lipids / TSH / microalbumin / A1C / UA, culture / PSA / iron studies / other:

DIAGNOSTICS XR / MRI / CT / US / cardiac / other
REFERRALS **F/U** ___ wk ___ mo

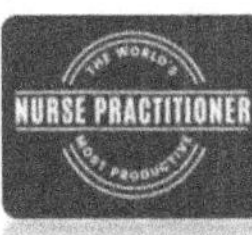

<table>
<tr><td>Patient ID#:
Reason for visit:</td><td>Date of visit:
Age: Gender:</td></tr>
</table>

BP: HT:
HR: WT:
T: BMI:
O2%:   PAIN:

NOTES . . . .

CONST Δ appetite, energy, weight / fever / chills / sweats / fatigue
HEAD trauma / mass / tenderness / rash / lesions
EYES visionΔ / itch / d/c / tears / dry / cataracts / glaucoma / glasses, contacts
ENT hearing Δ / pain / d/c / vertigo / ? infection // epistaxis / congestion // bleeding, swelling gums / pain / sore throat / voice Δ // neck pain / lumps / swelling / difficulty swallowing
CARDIAC pain / pressure / dizzy / N / orthopnea / edema / palp / weak w exertion / hx murmurs / hx MI / HTN / HF / numb / tingle / cold extrem / slow wound healing
RESP wheeze / SOB / cough / asthma / bronch / COPD
GI abd pain / Δ in bowels / constipation / diarrhea / N V / hepatitis / gallstones / dysphagia / reflux / hemorrhoids / black, bloody stools
GU burn / pain / nocturia / polyuria / hematuria / incontinence / infection / kid. stones
GENITAL DC / sores / pain / masses / last pap ______ / sexually active Y N / dyspareunia / LMP ______ / contraception
MSK redness / swelling / warmth / pain / +/- ROM / arthritis / musc cramps / fracture / sprains / joint replacement / stiffness: AM PM
SKIN rash / pruritis / jaundice / bruising / hx skin ca / mole Δ / Δ in hair, nails / lesions / slow wound healing
BREASTS lump / pain / dc / last mammo ______ / self exams YN
NEURO HA / seizure / vertigo / memory Δ / gait Δ / speech / coord
PSYCH depression / anxiety / Δ in sleep pattern / substance, ETOH abuse / suicidal ideation / homicidal ideation
ENDO polydipsia, polyuria / heat, cold intolerance / Δ hair/nails/energy
HEM/LYMPH anemia / bruising / hx transfusions / blood disorder / lymphadenopathy / axillary, groin tenderness
ALLX/IMMUN season allx / food allx / med allx / immune disorder:

SOCIAL HX # in household ______ / lives with SP/BF/GF/SO / children __ / tobacco Y/N #pk / sexual activity Y/N / etoh, other substances Y/N / occupation:
FAM HX ca / HTN / MI / CAD / stroke / hyperlipidemia / DM2 / Alzheimer's / depression / osteoporosis / other:

GENERAL well appearing / well nourished / a&o x 3 / normal mood / normal affect
NEURO intact / abnormal   **DTR:** 1 2 3 4 5 location:
SKIN + NAILS turgor / rash / bruising / lesions // texture, distribution of hair // nails: abnormal color / nail deformity
HEAD normocephalic / atraumatic / visible mass / palpable mass / depression / scarring
EYES acuity intact / conjunctiva clear / EOM intact / PERRLA / fundi: normal discs and vessels / icterus / exudate / hemorrhage
EARS EACs clear / TM translucent, mobile / landmarks abnormal / hearing diminished
NOSE lesions / mucosal inflammation / septum, turbinates abnormal / sinus tenderness
MOUTH mucous membranes dry / lesions / poor dentition / caries / gingival inflammation
PHARYNX mucosa inflammation / tonsillar hypertrophy / tonsillar exudate
NECK supple / ROM WNL / lesion / bruit / adenopathy / thyroid enlarged, tender / mass
CARDIAC regular rate, rhythm / S1, S2 / murmur / gallop / click / rub / PMI displacement
RESP clear to auscultation in all fields / wheezes (insp) (exp) / rales / crackles
ABDOMEN BSx4 / tender / organomegaly / mass / hernia
RECTAL abnormal tone / hemorrhoids (int/ext) / palpable mass
BACK abnormal curvature / tenderness / CVAT / Δ ROM
EXTREMITIES amputation / deformity / edema / varicosities / + pulses
MSK abnormal gait / asymmetry / crepitation / defect / tenderness / mass / effusion / Δ ROM / instability / atrophy / abnormal strength, tone in head, neck, spine, ribs, pelvis, UE, LE / pathologic reflexes
PSYCH A&O x3 / +recent/remote memory / insight / affect
BREAST nipple abnormality / mass / tenderness / axillary, clavicular adenopathy
GYN/GU lesions / d/c / uterus, adnexa tenderness / CMT // circumcised / penile lesions / urethra normal location, no d/c / testes normal / + cremasteric reflex
FEET + pulses / monofilament + / nails abnormal / dry, broken skin / callus

LABS CBC / CMP / lipids / TSH / microalbumin / A1C / UA, culture / PSA / iron studies / other:

DIAGNOSTICS XR / MRI / CT / US / cardiac / other
REFERRALS   **F/U** ___ wk ___ mo

<table>
<tr><td colspan="2"></td><td>BP:</td><td>HT:</td></tr>
<tr><td colspan="2">Patient ID#:   Date of visit:</td><td>HR:</td><td>WT:</td></tr>
<tr><td colspan="2">Reason for visit: Age: Gender:</td><td>T:</td><td>BMI:</td></tr>
<tr><td colspan="2"></td><td>O2%:</td><td>PAIN:</td></tr>
</table>

NOTES . . . .

CONST	Δ appetite, energy, weight / fever / chills / sweats / fatigue
HEAD	trauma / mass / tenderness / rash / lesions
EYES	visionΔ / itch / d/c / tears / dry / cataracts / glaucoma / glasses, contacts
ENT	hearing Δ / pain / d/c / vertigo / ? infection // epistaxis / congestion // bleeding, swelling gums / pain / sore throat / voice Δ // neck pain / lumps / swelling / difficulty swallowing
CARDIAC	pain / pressure / dizzy / N / orthopnea / edema / palp / weak w exertion / hx murmurs / hx MI / HTN / HF / numb / tingle / cold extrem / slow wound healing
RESP	wheeze / SOB / cough / asthma / bronch / COPD
GI	abd pain / Δ in bowels / constipation / diarrhea / N V / hepatitis / gallstones / dysphagia / reflux / hemorrhoids / black, bloody stools
GU	burn / pain / nocturia / polyuria / hematuria / incontinence / infection / kid. stones
GENITAL	DC / sores / pain / masses / last pap _______ / sexually active Y N / dyspareunia / LMP _______ / contraception
MSK	redness / swelling / warmth / pain / +/- ROM / arthritis / musc cramps / fracture / sprains / joint replacement / stiffness: AM PM
SKIN	rash / pruritis / jaundice / bruising / hx skin ca / mole Δ / Δ in hair, nails / lesions / slow wound healing
BREASTS	lump / pain / dc / last mammo _______ / self exams YN
NEURO	HA / seizure / vertigo / memory Δ / gait Δ / speech / coord
PSYCH	depression / anxiety / Δ in sleep pattern / substance, ETOH abuse / suicidal ideation / homicidal ideation
ENDO	polydipsia, polyuria / heat, cold intolerance / Δ hair/nails/energy
HEM/LYMPH	anemia / bruising / hx transfusions / blood disorder / lymphadenopathy / axillary, groin tenderness
ALLX/IMMUN	season allx / food allx / med allx / immune disorder:

SOCIAL HX	# in household _______ / lives with SP/BF/GF/SO / children __ / tobacco Y/N #pk / sexual activity Y/N / etoh, other substances Y/N / occupation:
FAM HX	ca / HTN / MI / CAD / stroke / hyperlipidemia / DM2 / Alzheimer's / depression / osteoporosis / other:

GENERAL	well appearing / well nourished / a&o x 3 / normal mood / normal affect
NEURO	intact / abnormal **DTR:** 1 2 3 4 5 location:
SKIN + NAILS	turgor / rash / bruising / lesions // texture, distribution of hair // nails: abnormal color / nail deformity
HEAD	normocephalic / atraumatic / visible mass / palpable mass / depression / scarring
EYES	acuity intact / conjunctiva clear / EOM intact / PERRLA / fundi: normal discs and vessels / icterus / exudate / hemorrhage
EARS	EACs clear / TM translucent, mobile / landmarks abnormal / hearing diminished
NOSE	lesions / mucosal inflammation / septum, turbinates abnormal / sinus tenderness
MOUTH	mucous membranes dry / lesions / poor dentition / caries / gingival inflammation
PHARYNX	mucosa inflammation / tonsillar hypertrophy / tonsillar exudate
NECK	supple / ROM WNL / lesion / bruit / adenopathy / thyroid enlarged, tender / mass
CARDIAC	regular rate, rhythm / S1, S2 / murmur / gallop / click / rub / PMI displacement
RESP	clear to auscultation in all fields / wheezes (insp) (exp) / rales / crackles
ABDOMEN	BSx4 / tender / organomegaly / mass / hernia
RECTAL	abnormal tone / hemorrhoids (int/ext) / palpable mass
BACK	abnormal curvature / tenderness / CVAT / Δ ROM
EXTREMITIES	amputation / deformity / edema / varicosities / + pulses
MSK	abnormal gait / asymmetry / crepitation / defect / tenderness / mass / effusion / Δ ROM / instability / atrophy / abnormal strength, tone in head, neck, spine, ribs, pelvis, UE, LE / pathologic reflexes
PSYCH	A&O x3 / +recent/remote memory / insight / affect
BREAST	nipple abnormality / mass / tenderness / axillary, clavicular adenopathy
GYN/GU	lesions / d/c / uterus, adnexa tenderness / CMT // circumcised / penile lesions / urethra normal location, no d/c / testes normal / + cremasteric reflex
FEET	+ pulses / monofilament + / nails abnormal / dry, broken skin / callus

LABS	CBC / CMP / lipids / TSH / microalbumin / A1C / UA, culture / PSA / iron studies / other:

DIAGNOSTICS	XR / MRI / CT / US / cardiac / other
REFERRALS	**F/U** ___ wk ___ mo

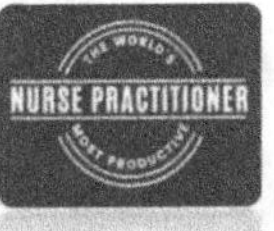

| Patient ID#: | Date of visit: |
| Reason for visit: | Age: Gender: |

BP: HT:
HR: WT:
T: BMI:
O2%:   PAIN:

NOTES . . . .

CONST Δ appetite, energy, weight / fever / chills / sweats / fatigue

HEAD trauma / mass / tenderness / rash / lesions

EYES visionΔ / itch / d/c / tears / dry / cataracts / glaucoma / glasses, contacts

ENT hearing Δ / pain / d/c / vertigo / ? infection // epistaxis / congestion // bleeding, swelling gums / pain / sore throat / voice Δ // neck pain / lumps / swelling / difficulty swallowing

CARDIAC pain / pressure / dizzy / N / orthopnea / edema / palp / weak w exertion / hx murmurs / hx MI / HTN / HF / numb / tingle / cold extrem / slow wound healing

RESP wheeze / SOB / cough / asthma / bronch / COPD

GI abd pain / Δ in bowels / constipation / diarrhea / N V / hepatitis / gallstones / dysphagia / reflux / hemorrhoids / black, bloody stools

GU burn / pain / nocturia / polyuria / hematuria / incontinence / infection / kid. stones

GENITAL DC / sores / pain / masses / last pap _____ / sexually active Y N / dyspareunia / LMP _______ / contraception

MSK redness / swelling / warmth / pain / +/- ROM / arthritis / musc cramps / fracture / sprains / joint replacement / stiffness: AM PM

SKIN rash / pruritis / jaundice / bruising / hx skin ca / mole Δ / Δ in hair, nails / lesions / slow wound healing

BREASTS lump / pain / dc / last mammo ____ / self exams YN

NEURO HA / seizure / vertigo / memory Δ / gait Δ / speech / coord

PSYCH depression / anxiety / Δ in sleep pattern / substance, ETOH abuse / suicidal ideation / homicidal ideation

ENDO polydipsia, polyuria / heat, cold intolerance / Δ hair/nails/energy

HEM/LYMPH anemia / bruising / hx transfusions / blood disorder / lymphadenopathy / axillary, groin tenderness

ALLX/IMMUN season allx / food allx / med allx / immune disorder:

SOCIAL HX # in household _____ / lives with SP/BF/GF/SO / children ___ / tobacco Y/N #pk / sexual activity Y/N / etoh, other substances Y/N / occupation:

FAM HX ca / HTN / MI / CAD / stroke / hyperlipidemia / DM2 / Alzheimer's / depression / osteoporosis / other:

GENERAL well appearing / well nourished / a&o x 3 / normal mood / normal affect

NEURO intact / abnormal   **DTR:** 1 2 3 4 5 location:

SKIN + NAILS turgor / rash / bruising / lesions // texture, distribution of hair // nails: abnormal color / nail deformity

HEAD normocephalic / atraumatic / visible mass / palpable mass / depression / scarring

EYES acuity intact / conjunctiva clear / EOM intact / PERRLA / fundi: normal discs and vessels / icterus / exudate / hemorrhage

EARS EACs clear / TM translucent, mobile / landmarks abnormal / hearing diminished

NOSE lesions / mucosal inflammation / septum, turbinates abnormal / sinus tenderness

MOUTH mucous membranes dry / lesions / poor dentition / caries / gingival inflammation

PHARYNX mucosa inflammation / tonsillar hypertrophy / tonsillar exudate

NECK supple / ROM WNL / lesion / bruit / adenopathy / thyroid enlarged, tender / mass

CARDIAC regular rate, rhythm / S1, S2 / murmur / gallop / click / rub / PMI displacement

RESP clear to auscultation in all fields / wheezes (insp) (exp) / rales / crackles

ABDOMEN BSx4 / tender / organomegaly / mass / hernia

RECTAL abnormal tone / hemorrhoids (int/ext) / palpable mass

BACK abnormal curvature / tenderness / CVAT / Δ ROM

EXTREMITIES amputation / deformity / edema / varicosities / + pulses

MSK abnormal gait / asymmetry / crepitation / defect / tenderness / mass / effusion / Δ ROM / instability / atrophy / abnormal strength, tone in head, neck, spine, ribs, pelvis, UE, LE / pathologic reflexes

PSYCH A&O x3 / +recent/remote memory / insight / affect

BREAST nipple abnormality / mass / tenderness / axillary, clavicular adenopathy

GYN/GU lesions / d/c / uterus, adnexa tenderness / CMT // circumcised / penile lesions / urethra normal location, no d/c / testes normal / + cremasteric reflex

FEET + pulses / monofilament + / nails abnormal / dry, broken skin / callus

---

LABS CBC / CMP / lipids / TSH / microalbumin / A1C / UA, culture / PSA / iron studies / other:

DIAGNOSTICS XR / MRI / CT / US / cardiac / other

REFERRALS   **F/U** ___ wk ___ mo

| Patient ID#: | Date of visit: |
| Reason for visit: | Age: Gender: |

BP: HT:
HR: WT:
T: BMI:
O2%:   PAIN:

NOTES . . . .

CONST Δ appetite, energy, weight / fever / chills / sweats / fatigue
HEAD trauma / mass / tenderness / rash / lesions
EYES visionΔ / itch / d/c / tears / dry / cataracts / glaucoma / glasses, contacts
ENT hearing Δ / pain / d/c / vertigo / ? infection // epistaxis / congestion // bleeding,
swelling gums / pain / sore throat / voice Δ // neck pain / lumps / swelling / difficulty
swallowing

CARDIAC pain / pressure / dizzy / N / orthopnea / edema / palp / weak w exertion / hx murmurs
/ hx MI / HTN / HF / numb / tingle / cold extrem / slow wound healing

RESP wheeze / SOB / cough / asthma / bronch / COPD
GI abd pain / Δ in bowels / constipation / diarrhea / N V / hepatitis / gallstones /
dysphagia / reflux / hemorrhoids / black, bloody stools

GU burn / pain / nocturia / polyuria / hematuria / incontinence / infection / kid. stones
GENITAL DC / sores / pain / masses / last pap _____ / sexually active Y N / dyspareunia /
LMP _______ / contraception

MSK redness / swelling / warmth / pain / +/- ROM / arthritis / musc cramps / fracture /
sprains / joint replacement / stiffness: AM PM

SKIN rash / pruritis / jaundice / bruising / hx skin ca / mole Δ / Δ in hair, nails / lesions /
slow wound healing

BREASTS lump / pain / dc / last mammo _______ / self exams YN
NEURO HA / seizure / vertigo / memory Δ / gait Δ / speech / coord
PSYCH depression / anxiety / Δ in sleep pattern / substance, ETOH abuse / suicidal ideation
/ homicidal ideation

ENDO polydipsia, polyuria / heat, cold intolerance / Δ hair/nails/energy
HEM/LYMPH anemia / bruising / hx transfusions / blood disorder / lymphadenopathy / axillary,
groin tenderness

ALLX/IMMUN season allx / food allx / med allx / immune disorder:

SOCIAL HX # in household _____ / lives with SP/BF/GF/SO / children __ / tobacco Y/N #pk /
sexual activity Y/N / etoh, other substances Y/N / occupation:

FAM HX ca / HTN / MI / CAD / stroke / hyperlipidemia / DM2 / Alzheimer's / depression /
osteoporosis / other:

GENERAL well appearing / well nourished / a&o x 3 / normal mood / normal affect
NEURO intact / abnormal   **DTR:** 1 2 3 4 5 location:
SKIN + NAILS turgor / rash / bruising / lesions // texture, distribution of hair // nails: abnormal color /
nail deformity

HEAD normocephalic / atraumatic / visible mass / palpable mass / depression / scarring
EYES acuity intact / conjunctiva clear / EOM intact / PERRLA / fundi: normal discs and
vessels / icterus / exudate / hemorrhage

EARS EACs clear / TM translucent, mobile / landmarks abnormal / hearing diminished
NOSE lesions / mucosal inflammation / septum, turbinates abnormal / sinus tenderness
MOUTH mucous membranes dry / lesions / poor dentition / caries / gingival inflammation
PHARYNX mucosa inflammation / tonsillar hypertrophy / tonsillar exudate
NECK supple / ROM WNL / lesion / bruit / adenopathy / thyroid enlarged, tender / mass
CARDIAC regular rate, rhythm / S1, S2 / murmur / gallop / click / rub / PMI displacement
RESP clear to auscultation in all fields / wheezes (insp) (exp) / rales / crackles
ABDOMEN BSx4 / tender / organomegaly / mass / hernia
RECTAL abnormal tone / hemorrhoids (int/ext) / palpable mass
BACK abnormal curvature / tenderness / CVAT / Δ ROM
EXTREMITIES amputation / deformity / edema / varicosities / + pulses
MSK abnormal gait / asymmetry / crepitation / defect / tenderness / mass / effusion / Δ
ROM / instability / atrophy / abnormal strength, tone in head, neck, spine, ribs,
pelvis, UE, LE / pathologic reflexes

PSYCH A&O x3 / +recent/remote memory / insight / affect
BREAST nipple abnormality / mass / tenderness / axillary, clavicular adenopathy
GYN/GU lesions / d/c / uterus, adnexa tenderness / CMT // circumcised / penile lesions /
urethra normal location, no d/c / testes normal / + cremasteric reflex
FEET + pulses / monofilament + / nails abnormal / dry, broken skin / callus

LABS CBC / CMP / lipids / TSH / microalbumin / A1C / UA, culture / PSA / iron studies /
other:

DIAGNOSTICS XR / MRI / CT / US / cardiac / other
REFERRALS   **F/U** ___ wk ___ mo

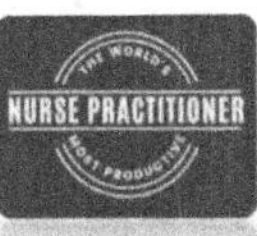

<table>
<tr><td colspan="2">

Patient ID#:

Reason for visit:
</td><td>

Date of visit:

Age: Gender:
</td></tr>
</table>

BP:	HT:
HR:	WT:
T:	BMI:
O2%:	PAIN:

NOTES . . . .

CONST	Δ appetite, energy, weight / fever / chills / sweats / fatigue
HEAD	trauma / mass / tenderness / rash / lesions
EYES	visionΔ / itch / d/c / tears / dry / cataracts / glaucoma / glasses, contacts
ENT	hearing Δ / pain / d/c / vertigo / ? infection // epistaxis / congestion // bleeding, swelling gums / pain / sore throat / voice Δ // neck pain / lumps / swelling / difficulty swallowing
CARDIAC	pain / pressure / dizzy / N / orthopnea / edema / palp / weak w exertion / hx murmurs / hx MI / HTN / HF / numb / tingle / cold extrem / slow wound healing
RESP	wheeze / SOB / cough / asthma / bronch / COPD
GI	abd pain / Δ in bowels / constipation / diarrhea / N V / hepatitis / gallstones / dysphagia / reflux / hemorrhoids / black, bloody stools
GU	burn / pain / nocturia / polyuria / hematuria / incontinence / infection / kid. stones
GENITAL	DC / sores / pain / masses / last pap ______ / sexually active Y N / dyspareunia / LMP ______ / contraception
MSK	redness / swelling / warmth / pain / +/- ROM / arthritis / musc cramps / fracture / sprains / joint replacement / stiffness: AM PM
SKIN	rash / pruritis / jaundice / bruising / hx skin ca / mole Δ / Δ in hair, nails / lesions / slow wound healing
BREASTS	lump / pain / dc / last mammo ______ / self exams YN
NEURO	HA / seizure / vertigo / memory Δ / gait Δ / speech / coord
PSYCH	depression / anxiety / Δ in sleep pattern / substance, ETOH abuse / suicidal ideation / homicidal ideation
ENDO	polydipsia, polyuria / heat, cold intolerance / Δ hair/nails/energy
HEM/LYMPH	anemia / bruising / hx transfusions / blood disorder / lymphadenopathy / axillary, groin tenderness
ALLX/IMMUN	season allx / food allx / med allx / immune disorder:

SOCIAL HX	# in household ______ / lives with SP/BF/GF/SO / children __ / tobacco Y/N #pk / sexual activity Y/N / etoh, other substances Y/N / occupation:
FAM HX	ca / HTN / MI / CAD / stroke / hyperlipidemia / DM2 / Alzheimer's / depression / osteoporosis / other:

GENERAL	well appearing / well nourished / a&o x 3 / normal mood / normal affect
NEURO	intact / abnormal **DTR:** 1 2 3 4 5 location:
SKIN + NAILS	turgor / rash / bruising / lesions // texture, distribution of hair // nails: abnormal color / nail deformity
HEAD	normocephalic / atraumatic / visible mass / palpable mass / depression / scarring
EYES	acuity intact / conjunctiva clear / EOM intact / PERRLA / fundi: normal discs and vessels / icterus / exudate / hemorrhage
EARS	EACs clear / TM translucent, mobile / landmarks abnormal / hearing diminished
NOSE	lesions / mucosal inflammation / septum, turbinates abnormal / sinus tenderness
MOUTH	mucous membranes dry / lesions / poor dentition / caries / gingival inflammation
PHARYNX	mucosa inflammation / tonsillar hypertrophy / tonsillar exudate
NECK	supple / ROM WNL / lesion / bruit / adenopathy / thyroid enlarged, tender / mass
CARDIAC	regular rate, rhythm / S1, S2 / murmur / gallop / click / rub / PMI displacement
RESP	clear to auscultation in all fields / wheezes (insp) (exp) / rales / crackles
ABDOMEN	BSx4 / tender / organomegaly / mass / hernia
RECTAL	abnormal tone / hemorrhoids (int/ext) / palpable mass
BACK	abnormal curvature / tenderness / CVAT / Δ ROM
EXTREMITIES	amputation / deformity / edema / varicosities / + pulses
MSK	abnormal gait / asymmetry / crepitation / defect / tenderness / mass / effusion / Δ ROM / instability / atrophy / abnormal strength, tone in head, neck, spine, ribs, pelvis, UE, LE / pathologic reflexes
PSYCH	A&O x3 / +recent/remote memory / insight / affect
BREAST	nipple abnormality / mass / tenderness / axillary, clavicular adenopathy
GYN/GU	lesions / d/c / uterus, adnexa tenderness / CMT // circumcised / penile lesions / urethra normal location, no d/c / testes normal / + cremasteric reflex
FEET	+ pulses / monofilament + / nails abnormal / dry, broken skin / callus

LABS	CBC / CMP / lipids / TSH / microalbumin / A1C / UA, culture / PSA / iron studies / other:

DIAGNOSTICS	XR / MRI / CT / US / cardiac / other
REFERRALS	**F/U** ___ wk ___ mo

<table>
<tr><td colspan="2">BP:</td><td>HT:</td></tr>
<tr><td colspan="2">HR:</td><td>WT:</td></tr>
<tr><td colspan="2">T:</td><td>BMI:</td></tr>
<tr><td colspan="2">O2%:</td><td>PAIN:</td></tr>
</table>

Patient ID#:	Date of visit:
Reason for visit:	Age: Gender:

NOTES . . . .

CONST	Δ appetite, energy, weight / fever / chills / sweats / fatigue
HEAD	trauma / mass / tenderness / rash / lesions
EYES	visionΔ / itch / d/c / tears / dry / cataracts / glaucoma / glasses, contacts
ENT	hearing Δ / pain / d/c / vertigo / ? infection // epistaxis / congestion // bleeding, swelling gums / pain / sore throat / voice Δ // neck pain / lumps / swelling / difficulty swallowing
CARDIAC	pain / pressure / dizzy / N / orthopnea / edema / palp / weak w exertion / hx murmurs / hx MI / HTN / HF / numb / tingle / cold extrem / slow wound healing
RESP	wheeze / SOB / cough / asthma / bronch / COPD
GI	abd pain / Δ in bowels / constipation / diarrhea / N V / hepatitis / gallstones / dysphagia / reflux / hemorrhoids / black, bloody stools
GU	burn / pain / nocturia / polyuria / hematuria / incontinence / infection / kid. stones
GENITAL	DC / sores / pain / masses / last pap ______ / sexually active Y N / dyspareunia / LMP ______ / contraception
MSK	redness / swelling / warmth / pain / +/- ROM / arthritis / musc cramps / fracture / sprains / joint replacement / stiffness: AM PM
SKIN	rash / pruritis / jaundice / bruising / hx skin ca / mole Δ / Δ in hair, nails / lesions / slow wound healing
BREASTS	lump / pain / dc / last mammo ______ / self exams YN
NEURO	HA / seizure / vertigo / memory Δ / gait Δ / speech / coord
PSYCH	depression / anxiety / Δ in sleep pattern / substance, ETOH abuse / suicidal ideation / homicidal ideation
ENDO	polydipsia, polyuria / heat, cold intolerance / Δ hair/nails/energy
HEM/LYMPH	anemia / bruising / hx transfusions / blood disorder / lymphadenopathy / axillary, groin tenderness
ALLX/IMMUN	season allx / food allx / med allx / immune disorder:

SOCIAL HX	# in household ______ / lives with SP/BF/GF/SO / children __ / tobacco Y/N #pk / sexual activity Y/N / etoh, other substances Y/N / occupation:
FAM HX	ca / HTN / MI / CAD / stroke / hyperlipidemia / DM2 / Alzheimer's / depression / osteoporosis / other:

GENERAL	well appearing / well nourished / a&o x 3 / normal mood / normal affect
NEURO	intact / abnormal **DTR:** 1 2 3 4 5 location:
SKIN + NAILS	turgor / rash / bruising / lesions // texture, distribution of hair // nails: abnormal color / nail deformity
HEAD	normocephalic / atraumatic / visible mass / palpable mass / depression / scarring
EYES	acuity intact / conjunctiva clear / EOM intact / PERRLA / fundi: normal discs and vessels / icterus / exudate / hemorrhage
EARS	EACs clear / TM translucent, mobile / landmarks abnormal / hearing diminished
NOSE	lesions / mucosal inflammation / septum, turbinates abnormal / sinus tenderness
MOUTH	mucous membranes dry / lesions / poor dentition / caries / gingival inflammation
PHARYNX	mucosa inflammation / tonsillar hypertrophy / tonsillar exudate
NECK	supple / ROM WNL / lesion / bruit / adenopathy / thyroid enlarged, tender / mass
CARDIAC	regular rate, rhythm / S1, S2 / murmur / gallop / click / rub / PMI displacement
RESP	clear to auscultation in all fields / wheezes (insp) (exp) / rales / crackles
ABDOMEN	BSx4 / tender / organomegaly / mass / hernia
RECTAL	abnormal tone / hemorrhoids (int/ext) / palpable mass
BACK	abnormal curvature / tenderness / CVAT / Δ ROM
EXTREMITIES	amputation / deformity / edema / varicosities / + pulses
MSK	abnormal gait / asymmetry / crepitation / defect / tenderness / mass / effusion / Δ ROM / instability / atrophy / abnormal strength, tone in head, neck, spine, ribs, pelvis, UE, LE / pathologic reflexes
PSYCH	A&O x3 / +recent/remote memory / insight / affect
BREAST	nipple abnormality / mass / tenderness / axillary, clavicular adenopathy
GYN/GU	lesions / d/c / uterus, adnexa tenderness / CMT // circumcised / penile lesions / urethra normal location, no d/c / testes normal / + cremasteric reflex
FEET	+ pulses / monofilament + / nails abnormal / dry, broken skin / callus

LABS	CBC / CMP / lipids / TSH / microalbumin / A1C / UA, culture / PSA / iron studies / other:

DIAGNOSTICS	XR / MRI / CT / US / cardiac / other
REFERRALS	**F/U** ___ wk ___ mo

<table>
<tr><td>Patient ID#:
Reason for visit:</td><td>Date of visit:
Age: Gender:</td></tr>
</table>

BP:	HT:
HR:	WT:
T:	BMI:
O2%:	PAIN:

NOTES . . . .

CONST	Δ appetite, energy, weight / fever / chills / sweats / fatigue
HEAD	trauma / mass / tenderness / rash / lesions
EYES	visionΔ / itch / d/c / tears / dry / cataracts / glaucoma / glasses, contacts
ENT	hearing Δ / pain / d/c / vertigo / ? infection // epistaxis / congestion // bleeding, swelling gums / pain / sore throat / voice Δ // neck pain / lumps / swelling / difficulty swallowing
CARDIAC	pain / pressure / dizzy / N / orthopnea / edema / palp / weak w exertion / hx murmurs / hx MI / HTN / HF / numb / tingle / cold extrem / slow wound healing
RESP	wheeze / SOB / cough / asthma / bronch / COPD
GI	abd pain / Δ in bowels / constipation / diarrhea / N V / hepatitis / gallstones / dysphagia / reflux / hemorrhoids / black, bloody stools
GU	burn / pain / nocturia / polyuria / hematuria / incontinence / infection / kid. stones
GENITAL	DC / sores / pain / masses / last pap ______ / sexually active Y N / dyspareunia / LMP ______ / contraception
MSK	redness / swelling / warmth / pain / +/- ROM / arthritis / musc cramps / fracture / sprains / joint replacement / stiffness: AM PM
SKIN	rash / pruritis / jaundice / bruising / hx skin ca / mole Δ / Δ in hair, nails / lesions / slow wound healing
BREASTS	lump / pain / dc / last mammo ______ / self exams YN
NEURO	HA / seizure / vertigo / memory Δ / gait Δ / speech / coord
PSYCH	depression / anxiety / Δ in sleep pattern / substance, ETOH abuse / suicidal ideation / homicidal ideation
ENDO	polydipsia, polyuria / heat, cold intolerance / Δ hair/nails/energy
HEM/LYMPH	anemia / bruising / hx transfusions / blood disorder / lymphadenopathy / axillary, groin tenderness
ALLX/IMMUN	season allx / food allx / med allx / immune disorder:

| **SOCIAL HX** | # in household ______ / lives with SP/BF/GF/SO / children __ / tobacco Y/N #pk / sexual activity Y/N / etoh, other substances Y/N / occupation: |
| **FAM HX** | ca / HTN / MI / CAD / stroke / hyperlipidemia / DM2 / Alzheimer's / depression / osteoporosis / other: |

GENERAL	well appearing / well nourished / a&o x 3 / normal mood / normal affect
NEURO	intact / abnormal **DTR:** 1 2 3 4 5 location:
SKIN + NAILS	turgor / rash / bruising / lesions // texture, distribution of hair // nails: abnormal color / nail deformity
HEAD	normocephalic / atraumatic / visible mass / palpable mass / depression / scarring
EYES	acuity intact / conjunctiva clear / EOM intact / PERRLA / fundi: normal discs and vessels / icterus / exudate / hemorrhage
EARS	EACs clear / TM translucent, mobile / landmarks abnormal / hearing diminished
NOSE	lesions / mucosal inflammation / septum, turbinates abnormal / sinus tenderness
MOUTH	mucous membranes dry / lesions / poor dentition / caries / gingival inflammation
PHARYNX	mucosa inflammation / tonsillar hypertrophy / tonsillar exudate
NECK	supple / ROM WNL / lesion / bruit / adenopathy / thyroid enlarged, tender / mass
CARDIAC	regular rate, rhythm / S1, S2 / murmur / gallop / click / rub / PMI displacement
RESP	clear to auscultation in all fields / wheezes (insp) (exp) / rales / crackles
ABDOMEN	BSx4 / tender / organomegaly / mass / hernia
RECTAL	abnormal tone / hemorrhoids (int/ext) / palpable mass
BACK	abnormal curvature / tenderness / CVAT / Δ ROM
EXTREMITIES	amputation / deformity / edema / varicosities / + pulses
MSK	abnormal gait / asymmetry / crepitation / defect / tenderness / mass / effusion / Δ ROM / instability / atrophy / abnormal strength, tone in head, neck, spine, ribs, pelvis, UE, LE / pathologic reflexes
PSYCH	A&O x3 / +recent/remote memory / insight / affect
BREAST	nipple abnormality / mass / tenderness / axillary, clavicular adenopathy
GYN/GU	lesions / d/c / uterus, adnexa tenderness / CMT // circumcised / penile lesions / urethra normal location, no d/c / testes normal / + cremasteric reflex
FEET	+ pulses / monofilament + / nails abnormal / dry, broken skin / callus

| **LABS** | CBC / CMP / lipids / TSH / microalbumin / A1C / UA, culture / PSA / iron studies / other: |

| **DIAGNOSTICS** | XR / MRI / CT / US / cardiac / other |
| **REFERRALS** | **F/U** ___ wk ___ mo |

<table>
<tr><td>Patient ID#:</td><td>Date of visit:</td></tr>
<tr><td>Reason for visit:</td><td>Age: Gender:</td></tr>
</table>

BP:	HT:
HR:	WT:
T:	BMI:
O2%:	PAIN:

NOTES . . . .

CONST — Δ appetite, energy, weight / fever / chills / sweats / fatigue
HEAD — trauma / mass / tenderness / rash / lesions
EYES — visionΔ / itch / d/c / tears / dry / cataracts / glaucoma / glasses, contacts
ENT — hearing Δ / pain / d/c / vertigo / ? infection // epistaxis / congestion // bleeding, swelling gums / pain / sore throat / voice Δ // neck pain / lumps / swelling / difficulty swallowing

CARDIAC — pain / pressure / dizzy / N / orthopnea / edema / palp / weak w exertion / hx murmurs / hx MI / HTN / HF / numb / tingle / cold extrem / slow wound healing
RESP — wheeze / SOB / cough / asthma / bronch / COPD
GI — abd pain / Δ in bowels / constipation / diarrhea / N V / hepatitis / gallstones / dysphagia / reflux / hemorrhoids / black, bloody stools
GU — burn / pain / nocturia / polyuria / hematuria / incontinence / infection / kid. stones
GENITAL — DC / sores / pain / masses / last pap _____ / sexually active Y N / dyspareunia / LMP _______ / contraception
MSK — redness / swelling / warmth / pain / +/- ROM / arthritis / musc cramps / fracture / sprains / joint replacement / stiffness: AM PM
SKIN — rash / pruritis / jaundice / bruising / hx skin ca / mole Δ / Δ in hair, nails / lesions / slow wound healing
BREASTS — lump / pain / dc / last mammo _______ / self exams YN
NEURO — HA / seizure / vertigo / memory Δ / gait Δ / speech / coord
PSYCH — depression / anxiety / Δ in sleep pattern / substance, ETOH abuse / suicidal ideation / homicidal ideation
ENDO — polydipsia, polyuria / heat, cold intolerance / Δ hair/nails/energy
HEM/LYMPH — anemia / bruising / hx transfusions / blood disorder / lymphadenopathy / axillary, groin tenderness
ALLX/IMMUN — season allx / food allx / med allx / immune disorder:

SOCIAL HX — # in household _____ / lives with SP/BF/GF/SO / children __ / tobacco Y/N #pk / sexual activity Y/N / etoh, other substances Y/N / occupation:
FAM HX — ca / HTN / MI / CAD / stroke / hyperlipidemia / DM2 / Alzheimer's / depression / osteoporosis / other:

GENERAL — well appearing / well nourished / a&o x 3 / normal mood / normal affect
NEURO — intact / abnormal   **DTR:** 1 2 3 4 5 location:
SKIN + NAILS — turgor / rash / bruising / lesions // texture, distribution of hair // nails: abnormal color / nail deformity
HEAD — normocephalic / atraumatic / visible mass / palpable mass / depression / scarring
EYES — acuity intact / conjunctiva clear / EOM intact / PERRLA / fundi: normal discs and vessels / icterus / exudate / hemorrhage
EARS — EACs clear / TM translucent, mobile / landmarks abnormal / hearing diminished
NOSE — lesions / mucosal inflammation / septum, turbinates abnormal / sinus tenderness
MOUTH — mucous membranes dry / lesions / poor dentition / caries / gingival inflammation
PHARYNX — mucosa inflammation / tonsillar hypertrophy / tonsillar exudate
NECK — supple / ROM WNL / lesion / bruit / adenopathy / thyroid enlarged, tender / mass
CARDIAC — regular rate, rhythm / S1, S2 / murmur / gallop / click / rub / PMI displacement
RESP — clear to auscultation in all fields / wheezes (insp) (exp) / rales / crackles
ABDOMEN — BSx4 / tender / organomegaly / mass / hernia
RECTAL — abnormal tone / hemorrhoids (int/ext) / palpable mass
BACK — abnormal curvature / tenderness / CVAT / Δ ROM
EXTREMITIES — amputation / deformity / edema / varicosities / + pulses
MSK — abnormal gait / asymmetry / crepitation / defect / tenderness / mass / effusion / Δ ROM / instability / atrophy / abnormal strength, tone in head, neck, spine, ribs, pelvis, UE, LE / pathologic reflexes
PSYCH — A&O x3 / +recent/remote memory / insight / affect
BREAST — nipple abnormality / mass / tenderness / axillary, clavicular adenopathy
GYN/GU — lesions / d/c / uterus, adnexa tenderness / CMT // circumcised / penile lesions / urethra normal location, no d/c / testes normal / + cremasteric reflex
FEET — + pulses / monofilament + / nails abnormal / dry, broken skin / callus

LABS — CBC / CMP / lipids / TSH / microalbumin / A1C / UA, culture / PSA / iron studies / other:

DIAGNOSTICS — XR / MRI / CT / US / cardiac / other
REFERRALS —   **F/U** ___ wk ___ mo

<table>
<tr><td colspan="2">Patient ID#:</td><td>Date of visit:</td></tr>
<tr><td colspan="2">Reason for visit:</td><td>Age: Gender:</td></tr>
</table>

<table>
<tr><td>BP:</td><td>HT:</td></tr>
<tr><td>HR:</td><td>WT:</td></tr>
<tr><td>T:</td><td>BMI:</td></tr>
<tr><td>O2%:</td><td>PAIN:</td></tr>
</table>

NOTES . . . .

CONST Δ appetite, energy, weight / fever / chills / sweats / fatigue

HEAD trauma / mass / tenderness / rash / lesions

EYES visionΔ / itch / d/c / tears / dry / cataracts / glaucoma / glasses, contacts

ENT hearing Δ / pain / d/c / vertigo / ? infection // epistaxis / congestion // bleeding, swelling gums / pain / sore throat / voice Δ // neck pain / lumps / swelling / difficulty swallowing

CARDIAC pain / pressure / dizzy / N / orthopnea / edema / palp / weak w exertion / hx murmurs / hx MI / HTN / HF / numb / tingle / cold extrem / slow wound healing

RESP wheeze / SOB / cough / asthma / bronch / COPD

GI abd pain / Δ in bowels / constipation / diarrhea / N V / hepatitis / gallstones / dysphagia / reflux / hemorrhoids / black, bloody stools

GU burn / pain / nocturia / polyuria / hematuria / incontinence / infection / kid. stones

GENITAL DC / sores / pain / masses / last pap ______ / sexually active Y N / dyspareunia / LMP ______ / contraception

MSK redness / swelling / warmth / pain / +/- ROM / arthritis / musc cramps / fracture / sprains / joint replacement / stiffness: AM PM

SKIN rash / pruritis / jaundice / bruising / hx skin ca / mole Δ / Δ in hair, nails / lesions / slow wound healing

BREASTS lump / pain / dc / last mammo ______ / self exams YN

NEURO HA / seizure / vertigo / memory Δ / gait Δ / speech / coord

PSYCH depression / anxiety / Δ in sleep pattern / substance, ETOH abuse / suicidal ideation / homicidal ideation

ENDO polydipsia, polyuria / heat, cold intolerance / Δ hair/nails/energy

HEM/LYMPH anemia / bruising / hx transfusions / blood disorder / lymphadenopathy / axillary, groin tenderness

ALLX/IMMUN season allx / food allx / med allx / immune disorder:

SOCIAL HX # in household ______ / lives with SP/BF/GF/SO / children __ / tobacco Y/N #pk / sexual activity Y/N / etoh, other substances Y/N / occupation:

FAM HX ca / HTN / MI / CAD / stroke / hyperlipidemia / DM2 / Alzheimer's / depression / osteoporosis / other:

GENERAL well appearing / well nourished / a&o x 3 / normal mood / normal affect

NEURO intact / abnormal   **DTR:** 1 2 3 4 5 location:

SKIN + NAILS turgor / rash / bruising / lesions // texture, distribution of hair // nails: abnormal color / nail deformity

HEAD normocephalic / atraumatic / visible mass / palpable mass / depression / scarring

EYES acuity intact / conjunctiva clear / EOM intact / PERRLA / fundi: normal discs and vessels / icterus / exudate / hemorrhage

EARS EACs clear / TM translucent, mobile / landmarks abnormal / hearing diminished

NOSE lesions / mucosal inflammation / septum, turbinates abnormal / sinus tenderness

MOUTH mucous membranes dry / lesions / poor dentition / caries / gingival inflammation

PHARYNX mucosa inflammation / tonsillar hypertrophy / tonsillar exudate

NECK supple / ROM WNL / lesion / bruit / adenopathy / thyroid enlarged, tender / mass

CARDIAC regular rate, rhythm / S1, S2 / murmur / gallop / click / rub / PMI displacement

RESP clear to auscultation in all fields / wheezes (insp) (exp) / rales / crackles

ABDOMEN BSx4 / tender / organomegaly / mass / hernia

RECTAL abnormal tone / hemorrhoids (int/ext) / palpable mass

BACK abnormal curvature / tenderness / CVAT / Δ ROM

EXTREMITIES amputation / deformity / edema / varicosities / + pulses

MSK abnormal gait / asymmetry / crepitation / defect / tenderness / mass / effusion / Δ ROM / instability / atrophy / abnormal strength, tone in head, neck, spine, ribs, pelvis, UE, LE / pathologic reflexes

PSYCH A&O x3 / +recent/remote memory / insight / affect

BREAST nipple abnormality / mass / tenderness / axillary, clavicular adenopathy

GYN/GU lesions / d/c / uterus, adnexa tenderness / CMT // circumcised / penile lesions / urethra normal location, no d/c / testes normal / + cremasteric reflex

FEET + pulses / monofilament + / nails abnormal / dry, broken skin / callus

LABS CBC / CMP / lipids / TSH / microalbumin / A1C / UA, culture / PSA / iron studies / other:

DIAGNOSTICS XR / MRI / CT / US / cardiac / other

REFERRALS   **F/U** ___ wk ___ mo

<table>
<tr><td colspan="2">

Patient ID#:
Reason for visit:

</td><td>

Date of visit:
Age: Gender:

</td></tr>
</table>

BP: HT:
HR: WT:
T: BMI:
O2%:   PAIN:

NOTES . . . .

CONST	Δ appetite, energy, weight / fever / chills / sweats / fatigue
HEAD	trauma / mass / tenderness / rash / lesions
EYES	visionΔ / itch / d/c / tears / dry / cataracts / glaucoma / glasses, contacts
ENT	hearing Δ / pain / d/c / vertigo / ? infection // epistaxis / congestion // bleeding, swelling gums / pain / sore throat / voice Δ // neck pain / lumps / swelling / difficulty swallowing
CARDIAC	pain / pressure / dizzy / N / orthopnea / edema / palp / weak w exertion / hx murmurs / hx MI / HTN / HF / numb / tingle / cold extrem / slow wound healing
RESP	wheeze / SOB / cough / asthma / bronch / COPD
GI	abd pain / Δ in bowels / constipation / diarrhea / N V / hepatitis / gallstones / dysphagia / reflux / hemorrhoids / black, bloody stools
GU	burn / pain / nocturia / polyuria / hematuria / incontinence / infection / kid. stones
GENITAL	DC / sores / pain / masses / last pap ______ / sexually active Y N / dyspareunia / LMP ______ / contraception
MSK	redness / swelling / warmth / pain / +/- ROM / arthritis / musc cramps / fracture / sprains / joint replacement / stiffness: AM PM
SKIN	rash / pruritis / jaundice / bruising / hx skin ca / mole Δ / Δ in hair, nails / lesions / slow wound healing
BREASTS	lump / pain / dc / last mammo ______ / self exams YN
NEURO	HA / seizure / vertigo / memory Δ / gait Δ / speech / coord
PSYCH	depression / anxiety / Δ in sleep pattern / substance, ETOH abuse / suicidal ideation / homicidal ideation
ENDO	polydipsia, polyuria / heat, cold intolerance / Δ hair/nails/energy
HEM/LYMPH	anemia / bruising / hx transfusions / blood disorder / lymphadenopathy / axillary, groin tenderness
ALLX/IMMUN	season allx / food allx / med allx / immune disorder:

SOCIAL HX	# in household ______ / lives with SP/BF/GF/SO / children __ / tobacco Y/N #pk / sexual activity Y/N / etoh, other substances Y/N / occupation:
FAM HX	ca / HTN / MI / CAD / stroke / hyperlipidemia / DM2 / Alzheimer's / depression / osteoporosis / other:

GENERAL	well appearing / well nourished / a&o x 3 / normal mood / normal affect
NEURO	intact / abnormal **DTR:** 1 2 3 4 5 location:
SKIN + NAILS	turgor / rash / bruising / lesions // texture, distribution of hair // nails: abnormal color / nail deformity
HEAD	normocephalic / atraumatic / visible mass / palpable mass / depression / scarring
EYES	acuity intact / conjunctiva clear / EOM intact / PERRLA / fundi: normal discs and vessels / icterus / exudate / hemorrhage
EARS	EACs clear / TM translucent, mobile / landmarks abnormal / hearing diminished
NOSE	lesions / mucosal inflammation / septum, turbinates abnormal / sinus tenderness
MOUTH	mucous membranes dry / lesions / poor dentition / caries / gingival inflammation
PHARYNX	mucosa inflammation / tonsillar hypertrophy / tonsillar exudate
NECK	supple / ROM WNL / lesion / bruit / adenopathy / thyroid enlarged, tender / mass
CARDIAC	regular rate, rhythm / S1, S2 / murmur / gallop / click / rub / PMI displacement
RESP	clear to auscultation in all fields / wheezes (insp) (exp) / rales / crackles
ABDOMEN	BSx4 / tender / organomegaly / mass / hernia
RECTAL	abnormal tone / hemorrhoids (int/ext) / palpable mass
BACK	abnormal curvature / tenderness / CVAT / Δ ROM
EXTREMITIES	amputation / deformity / edema / varicosities / + pulses
MSK	abnormal gait / asymmetry / crepitation / defect / tenderness / mass / effusion / Δ ROM / instability / atrophy / abnormal strength, tone in head, neck, spine, ribs, pelvis, UE, LE / pathologic reflexes
PSYCH	A&O x3 / +recent/remote memory / insight / affect
BREAST	nipple abnormality / mass / tenderness / axillary, clavicular adenopathy
GYN/GU	lesions / d/c / uterus, adnexa tenderness / CMT // circumcised / penile lesions / urethra normal location, no d/c / testes normal / + cremasteric reflex
FEET	+ pulses / monofilament + / nails abnormal / dry, broken skin / callus

LABS	CBC / CMP / lipids / TSH / microalbumin / A1C / UA, culture / PSA / iron studies / other:

DIAGNOSTICS	XR / MRI / CT / US / cardiac / other
REFERRALS	**F/U** ___ wk ___ mo

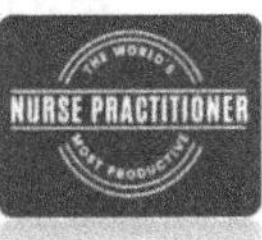

| Patient ID#: | Date of visit: |
| Reason for visit: | Age: Gender: |

BP: HT:
HR: WT:
T: BMI:
O2%:   PAIN:

CONST	Δ appetite, energy, weight / fever / chills / sweats / fatigue
HEAD	trauma / mass / tenderness / rash / lesions
EYES	visionΔ / itch / d/c / tears / dry / cataracts / glaucoma / glasses, contacts
ENT	hearing Δ / pain / d/c / vertigo / ? infection // epistaxis / congestion // bleeding, swelling gums / pain / sore throat / voice Δ // neck pain / lumps / swelling / difficulty swallowing
CARDIAC	pain / pressure / dizzy / N / orthopnea / edema / palp / weak w exertion / hx murmurs / hx MI / HTN / HF / numb / tingle / cold extrem / slow wound healing
RESP	wheeze / SOB / cough / asthma / bronch / COPD
GI	abd pain / Δ in bowels / constipation / diarrhea / N V / hepatitis / gallstones / dysphagia / reflux / hemorrhoids / black, bloody stools
GU	burn / pain / nocturia / polyuria / hematuria / incontinence / infection / kid. stones
GENITAL	DC / sores / pain / masses / last pap _____ / sexually active Y N / dyspareunia / LMP ______ / contraception
MSK	redness / swelling / warmth / pain / +/- ROM / arthritis / musc cramps / fracture / sprains / joint replacement / stiffness: AM PM
SKIN	rash / pruritis / jaundice / bruising / hx skin ca / mole Δ / Δ in hair, nails / lesions / slow wound healing
BREASTS	lump / pain / dc / last mammo _____ / self exams YN
NEURO	HA / seizure / vertigo / memory Δ / gait Δ / speech / coord
PSYCH	depression / anxiety / Δ in sleep pattern / substance, ETOH abuse / suicidal ideation / homicidal ideation
ENDO	polydipsia, polyuria / heat, cold intolerance / Δ hair/nails/energy
HEM/LYMPH	anemia / bruising / hx transfusions / blood disorder / lymphadenopathy / axillary, groin tenderness
ALLX/IMMUN	season allx / food allx / med allx / immune disorder:

SOCIAL HX	# in household _____ / lives with SP/BF/GF/SO / children __ / tobacco Y/N #pk / sexual activity Y/N / etoh, other substances Y/N / occupation:
FAM HX	ca / HTN / MI / CAD / stroke / hyperlipidemia / DM2 / Alzheimer's / depression / osteoporosis / other:

GENERAL	well appearing / well nourished / a&o x 3 / normal mood / normal affect
NEURO	intact / abnormal **DTR:** 1 2 3 4 5 location:
SKIN + NAILS	turgor / rash / bruising / lesions // texture, distribution of hair // nails: abnormal color / nail deformity
HEAD	normocephalic / atraumatic / visible mass / palpable mass / depression / scarring
EYES	acuity intact / conjunctiva clear / EOM intact / PERRLA / fundi: normal discs and vessels / icterus / exudate / hemorrhage
EARS	EACs clear / TM translucent, mobile / landmarks abnormal / hearing diminished
NOSE	lesions / mucosal inflammation / septum, turbinates abnormal / sinus tenderness
MOUTH	mucous membranes dry / lesions / poor dentition / caries / gingival inflammation
PHARYNX	mucosa inflammation / tonsillar hypertrophy / tonsillar exudate
NECK	supple / ROM WNL / lesion / bruit / adenopathy / thyroid enlarged, tender / mass
CARDIAC	regular rate, rhythm / S1, S2 / murmur / gallop / click / rub / PMI displacement
RESP	clear to auscultation in all fields / wheezes (insp) (exp) / rales / crackles
ABDOMEN	BSx4 / tender / organomegaly / mass / hernia
RECTAL	abnormal tone / hemorrhoids (int/ext) / palpable mass
BACK	abnormal curvature / tenderness / CVAT / Δ ROM
EXTREMITIES	amputation / deformity / edema / varicosities / + pulses
MSK	abnormal gait / asymmetry / crepitation / defect / tenderness / mass / effusion / Δ ROM / instability / atrophy / abnormal strength, tone in head, neck, spine, ribs, pelvis, UE, LE / pathologic reflexes
PSYCH	A&O x3 / +recent/remote memory / insight / affect
BREAST	nipple abnormality / mass / tenderness / axillary, clavicular adenopathy
GYN/GU	lesions / d/c / uterus, adnexa tenderness / CMT // circumcised / penile lesions / urethra normal location, no d/c / testes normal / + cremasteric reflex
FEET	+ pulses / monofilament + / nails abnormal / dry, broken skin / callus

LABS	CBC / CMP / lipids / TSH / microalbumin / A1C / UA, culture / PSA / iron studies / other:

DIAGNOSTICS	XR / MRI / CT / US / cardiac / other
REFERRALS	**F/U** ___ wk ___ mo

<table>
<tr><td colspan="2" style="border:1px solid black">

Patient ID#:

Reason for visit:
</td><td colspan="2">

Date of visit:

Age: Gender:
</td></tr>
</table>

BP:	**HT:**
HR:	**WT:**
T:	**BMI:**
O2%:	**PAIN:**

NOTES . . . .

CONST	Δ appetite, energy, weight / fever / chills / sweats / fatigue
HEAD	trauma / mass / tenderness / rash / lesions
EYES	visionΔ / itch / d/c / tears / dry / cataracts / glaucoma / glasses, contacts
ENT	hearing Δ / pain / d/c / vertigo / ? infection // epistaxis / congestion // bleeding, swelling gums / pain / sore throat / voice Δ // neck pain / lumps / swelling / difficulty swallowing
CARDIAC	pain / pressure / dizzy / N / orthopnea / edema / palp / weak w exertion / hx murmurs / hx MI / HTN / HF / numb / tingle / cold extrem / slow wound healing
RESP	wheeze / SOB / cough / asthma / bronch / COPD
GI	abd pain / Δ in bowels / constipation / diarrhea / N V / hepatitis / gallstones / dysphagia / reflux / hemorrhoids / black, bloody stools
GU	burn / pain / nocturia / polyuria / hematuria / incontinence / infection / kid. stones
GENITAL	DC / sores / pain / masses / last pap _____ / sexually active Y N / dyspareunia / LMP _____ / contraception
MSK	redness / swelling / warmth / pain / +/- ROM / arthritis / musc cramps / fracture / sprains / joint replacement / stiffness: AM PM
SKIN	rash / pruritis / jaundice / bruising / hx skin ca / mole Δ / Δ in hair, nails / lesions / slow wound healing
BREASTS	lump / pain / dc / last mammo _____ / self exams YN
NEURO	HA / seizure / vertigo / memory Δ / gait Δ / speech / coord
PSYCH	depression / anxiety / Δ in sleep pattern / substance, ETOH abuse / suicidal ideation / homicidal ideation
ENDO	polydipsia, polyuria / heat, cold intolerance / Δ hair/nails/energy
HEM/LYMPH	anemia / bruising / hx transfusions / blood disorder / lymphadenopathy / axillary, groin tenderness
ALLX/IMMUN	season allx / food allx / med allx / immune disorder:
SOCIAL HX	# in household _____ / lives with SP/BF/GF/SO / children __ / tobacco Y/N #pk / sexual activity Y/N / etoh, other substances Y/N / occupation:
FAM HX	ca / HTN / MI / CAD / stroke / hyperlipidemia / DM2 / Alzheimer's / depression / osteoporosis / other:
GENERAL	well appearing / well nourished / a&o x 3 / normal mood / normal affect
NEURO	intact / abnormal **DTR:** 1 2 3 4 5 location:
SKIN + NAILS	turgor / rash / bruising / lesions // texture, distribution of hair // nails: abnormal color / nail deformity
HEAD	normocephalic / atraumatic / visible mass / palpable mass / depression / scarring
EYES	acuity intact / conjunctiva clear / EOM intact / PERRLA / fundi: normal discs and vessels / icterus / exudate / hemorrhage
EARS	EACs clear / TM translucent, mobile / landmarks abnormal / hearing diminished
NOSE	lesions / mucosal inflammation / septum, turbinates abnormal / sinus tenderness
MOUTH	mucous membranes dry / lesions / poor dentition / caries / gingival inflammation
PHARYNX	mucosa inflammation / tonsillar hypertrophy / tonsillar exudate
NECK	supple / ROM WNL / lesion / bruit / adenopathy / thyroid enlarged, tender / mass
CARDIAC	regular rate, rhythm / S1, S2 / murmur / gallop / click / rub / PMI displacement
RESP	clear to auscultation in all fields / wheezes (insp) (exp) / rales / crackles
ABDOMEN	BSx4 / tender / organomegaly / mass / hernia
RECTAL	abnormal tone / hemorrhoids (int/ext) / palpable mass
BACK	abnormal curvature / tenderness / CVAT / Δ ROM
EXTREMITIES	amputation / deformity / edema / varicosities / + pulses
MSK	abnormal gait / asymmetry / crepitation / defect / tenderness / mass / effusion / Δ ROM / instability / atrophy / abnormal strength, tone in head, neck, spine, ribs, pelvis, UE, LE / pathologic reflexes
PSYCH	A&O x3 / +recent/remote memory / insight / affect
BREAST	nipple abnormality / mass / tenderness / axillary, clavicular adenopathy
GYN/GU	lesions / d/c / uterus, adnexa tenderness / CMT // circumcised / penile lesions / urethra normal location, no d/c / testes normal / + cremasteric reflex
FEET	+ pulses / monofilament + / nails abnormal / dry, broken skin / callus
LABS	CBC / CMP / lipids / TSH / microalbumin / A1C / UA, culture / PSA / iron studies / other:
DIAGNOSTICS	XR / MRI / CT / US / cardiac / other
REFERRALS	**F/U** ___ wk ___ mo

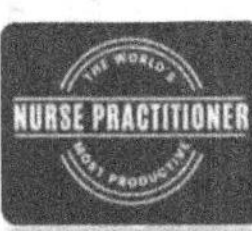

<table>
<tr><td colspan="2">

Patient ID#:
Reason for visit:
</td><td colspan="2">

Date of visit:
Age: **Gender:**
</td></tr>
</table>

BP: **HT:**
HR: **WT:**
T: **BMI:**
O2%:   **PAIN:**

NOTES . . . .

CONST	Δ appetite, energy, weight / fever / chills / sweats / fatigue
HEAD	trauma / mass / tenderness / rash / lesions
EYES	visionΔ / itch / d/c / tears / dry / cataracts / glaucoma / glasses, contacts
ENT	hearing Δ / pain / d/c / vertigo / ? infection // epistaxis / congestion // bleeding, swelling gums / pain / sore throat / voice Δ // neck pain / lumps / swelling / difficulty swallowing
CARDIAC	pain / pressure / dizzy / N / orthopnea / edema / palp / weak w exertion / hx murmurs / hx MI / HTN / HF / numb / tingle / cold extrem / slow wound healing
RESP	wheeze / SOB / cough / asthma / bronch / COPD
GI	abd pain / Δ in bowels / constipation / diarrhea / N V / hepatitis / gallstones / dysphagia / reflux / hemorrhoids / black, bloody stools
GU	burn / pain / nocturia / polyuria / hematuria / incontinence / infection / kid. stones
GENITAL	DC / sores / pain / masses / last pap _______ / sexually active Y N / dyspareunia / LMP _______ / contraception
MSK	redness / swelling / warmth / pain / +/- ROM / arthritis / musc cramps / fracture / sprains / joint replacement / stiffness: AM PM
SKIN	rash / pruritis / jaundice / bruising / hx skin ca / mole Δ / Δ in hair, nails / lesions / slow wound healing
BREASTS	lump / pain / dc / last mammo _______ / self exams YN
NEURO	HA / seizure / vertigo / memory Δ / gait Δ / speech / coord
PSYCH	depression / anxiety / Δ in sleep pattern / substance, ETOH abuse / suicidal ideation / homicidal ideation
ENDO	polydipsia, polyuria / heat, cold intolerance / Δ hair/nails/energy
HEM/LYMPH	anemia / bruising / hx transfusions / blood disorder / lymphadenopathy / axillary, groin tenderness
ALLX/IMMUN	season allx / food allx / med allx / immune disorder:

SOCIAL HX	# in household _______ / lives with SP/BF/GF/SO / children __ / tobacco Y/N #pk / sexual activity Y/N / etoh, other substances Y/N / occupation:
FAM HX	ca / HTN / MI / CAD / stroke / hyperlipidemia / DM2 / Alzheimer's / depression / osteoporosis / other:

GENERAL	well appearing / well nourished / a&o x 3 / normal mood / normal affect
NEURO	intact / abnormal **DTR:** 1 2 3 4 5 location:
SKIN + NAILS	turgor / rash / bruising / lesions // texture, distribution of hair // nails: abnormal color / nail deformity
HEAD	normocephalic / atraumatic / visible mass / palpable mass / depression / scarring
EYES	acuity intact / conjunctiva clear / EOM intact / PERRLA / fundi: normal discs and vessels / icterus / exudate / hemorrhage
EARS	EACs clear / TM translucent, mobile / landmarks abnormal / hearing diminished
NOSE	lesions / mucosal inflammation / septum, turbinates abnormal / sinus tenderness
MOUTH	mucous membranes dry / lesions / poor dentition / caries / gingival inflammation
PHARYNX	mucosa inflammation / tonsillar hypertrophy / tonsillar exudate
NECK	supple / ROM WNL / lesion / bruit / adenopathy / thyroid enlarged, tender / mass
CARDIAC	regular rate, rhythm / S1, S2 / murmur / gallop / click / rub / PMI displacement
RESP	clear to auscultation in all fields / wheezes (insp) (exp) / rales / crackles
ABDOMEN	BSx4 / tender / organomegaly / mass / hernia
RECTAL	abnormal tone / hemorrhoids (int/ext) / palpable mass
BACK	abnormal curvature / tenderness / CVAT / Δ ROM
EXTREMITIES	amputation / deformity / edema / varicosities / + pulses
MSK	abnormal gait / asymmetry / crepitation / defect / tenderness / mass / effusion / Δ ROM / instability / atrophy / abnormal strength, tone in head, neck, spine, ribs, pelvis, UE, LE / pathologic reflexes
PSYCH	A&O x3 / +recent/remote memory / insight / affect
BREAST	nipple abnormality / mass / tenderness / axillary, clavicular adenopathy
GYN/GU	lesions / d/c / uterus, adnexa tenderness / CMT // circumcised / penile lesions / urethra normal location, no d/c / testes normal / + cremasteric reflex
FEET	+ pulses / monofilament + / nails abnormal / dry, broken skin / callus

LABS	CBC / CMP / lipids / TSH / microalbumin / A1C / UA, culture / PSA / iron studies / other:

DIAGNOSTICS	XR / MRI / CT / US / cardiac / other
REFERRALS	**F/U** ___ wk ___ mo

| Patient ID#: | Date of visit: |
| Reason for visit: | Age: Gender: |

BP: HT:
HR: WT:
T: BMI:
O2%:   PAIN:

NOTES . . . .

CONST	Δ appetite, energy, weight / fever / chills / sweats / fatigue
HEAD	trauma / mass / tenderness / rash / lesions
EYES	visionΔ / itch / d/c / tears / dry / cataracts / glaucoma / glasses, contacts
ENT	hearing Δ / pain / d/c / vertigo / ? infection // epistaxis / congestion // bleeding, swelling gums / pain / sore throat / voice Δ // neck pain / lumps / swelling / difficulty swallowing
CARDIAC	pain / pressure / dizzy / N / orthopnea / edema / palp / weak w exertion / hx murmurs / hx MI / HTN / HF / numb / tingle / cold extrem / slow wound healing
RESP	wheeze / SOB / cough / asthma / bronch / COPD
GI	abd pain / Δ in bowels / constipation / diarrhea / N V / hepatitis / gallstones / dysphagia / reflux / hemorrhoids / black, bloody stools
GU	burn / pain / nocturia / polyuria / hematuria / incontinence / infection / kid. stones
GENITAL	DC / sores / pain / masses / last pap _____ / sexually active Y N / dyspareunia / LMP _____ / contraception
MSK	redness / swelling / warmth / pain / +/- ROM / arthritis / musc cramps / fracture / sprains / joint replacement / stiffness: AM PM
SKIN	rash / pruritis / jaundice / bruising / hx skin ca / mole Δ / Δ in hair, nails / lesions / slow wound healing
BREASTS	lump / pain / dc / last mammo _____ / self exams YN
NEURO	HA / seizure / vertigo / memory Δ / gait Δ / speech / coord
PSYCH	depression / anxiety / Δ in sleep pattern / substance, ETOH abuse / suicidal ideation / homicidal ideation
ENDO	polydipsia, polyuria / heat, cold intolerance / Δ hair/nails/energy
HEM/LYMPH	anemia / bruising / hx transfusions / blood disorder / lymphadenopathy / axillary, groin tenderness
ALLX/IMMUN	season allx / food allx / med allx / immune disorder:

SOCIAL HX	# in household _____ / lives with SP/BF/GF/SO / children __ / tobacco Y/N #pk / sexual activity Y/N / etoh, other substances Y/N / occupation:
FAM HX	ca / HTN / MI / CAD / stroke / hyperlipidemia / DM2 / Alzheimer's / depression / osteoporosis / other:

GENERAL	well appearing / well nourished / a&o x 3 / normal mood / normal affect
NEURO	intact / abnormal **DTR:** 1 2 3 4 5 location:
SKIN + NAILS	turgor / rash / bruising / lesions // texture, distribution of hair // nails: abnormal color / nail deformity
HEAD	normocephalic / atraumatic / visible mass / palpable mass / depression / scarring
EYES	acuity intact / conjunctiva clear / EOM intact / PERRLA / fundi: normal discs and vessels / icterus / exudate / hemorrhage
EARS	EACs clear / TM translucent, mobile / landmarks abnormal / hearing diminished
NOSE	lesions / mucosal inflammation / septum, turbinates abnormal / sinus tenderness
MOUTH	mucous membranes dry / lesions / poor dentition / caries / gingival inflammation
PHARYNX	mucosa inflammation / tonsillar hypertrophy / tonsillar exudate
NECK	supple / ROM WNL / lesion / bruit / adenopathy / thyroid enlarged, tender / mass
CARDIAC	regular rate, rhythm / S1, S2 / murmur / gallop / click / rub / PMI displacement
RESP	clear to auscultation in all fields / wheezes (insp) (exp) / rales / crackles
ABDOMEN	BSx4 / tender / organomegaly / mass / hernia
RECTAL	abnormal tone / hemorrhoids (int/ext) / palpable mass
BACK	abnormal curvature / tenderness / CVAT / Δ ROM
EXTREMITIES	amputation / deformity / edema / varicosities / + pulses
MSK	abnormal gait / asymmetry / crepitation / defect / tenderness / mass / effusion / Δ ROM / instability / atrophy / abnormal strength, tone in head, neck, spine, ribs, pelvis, UE, LE / pathologic reflexes
PSYCH	A&O x3 / +recent/remote memory / insight / affect
BREAST	nipple abnormality / mass / tenderness / axillary, clavicular adenopathy
GYN/GU	lesions / d/c / uterus, adnexa tenderness / CMT // circumcised / penile lesions / urethra normal location, no d/c / testes normal / + cremasteric reflex
FEET	+ pulses / monofilament + / nails abnormal / dry, broken skin / callus

LABS	CBC / CMP / lipids / TSH / microalbumin / A1C / UA, culture / PSA / iron studies / other:
DIAGNOSTICS	XR / MRI / CT / US / cardiac / other
REFERRALS	**F/U** ___ wk ___ mo

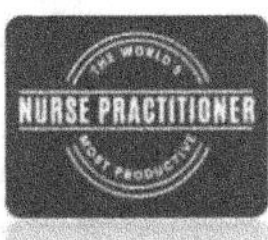

<table>
<tr><td>

Patient ID#:
Reason for visit:

Date of visit:
Age: Gender:

</td><td>

BP: HT:
HR: WT:
T: BMI:
O2%:   PAIN:

NOTES . . . .

</td></tr>
</table>

CONST	Δ appetite, energy, weight / fever / chills / sweats / fatigue
HEAD	trauma / mass / tenderness / rash / lesions
EYES	visionΔ / itch / d/c / tears / dry / cataracts / glaucoma / glasses, contacts
ENT	hearing Δ / pain / d/c / vertigo / ? infection // epistaxis / congestion // bleeding, swelling gums / pain / sore throat / voice Δ // neck pain / lumps / swelling / difficulty swallowing
CARDIAC	pain / pressure / dizzy / N / orthopnea / edema / palp / weak w exertion / hx murmurs / hx MI / HTN / HF / numb / tingle / cold extrem / slow wound healing
RESP	wheeze / SOB / cough / asthma / bronch / COPD
GI	abd pain / Δ in bowels / constipation / diarrhea / N V / hepatitis / gallstones / dysphagia / reflux / hemorrhoids / black, bloody stools
GU	burn / pain / nocturia / polyuria / hematuria / incontinence / infection / kid. stones
GENITAL	DC / sores / pain / masses / last pap ______ / sexually active Y N / dyspareunia / LMP ______ / contraception
MSK	redness / swelling / warmth / pain / +/- ROM / arthritis / musc cramps / fracture / sprains / joint replacement / stiffness: AM PM
SKIN	rash / pruritis / jaundice / bruising / hx skin ca / mole Δ / Δ in hair, nails / lesions / slow wound healing
BREASTS	lump / pain / dc / last mammo ______ / self exams YN
NEURO	HA / seizure / vertigo / memory Δ / gait Δ / speech / coord
PSYCH	depression / anxiety / Δ in sleep pattern / substance, ETOH abuse / suicidal ideation / homicidal ideation
ENDO	polydipsia, polyuria / heat, cold intolerance / Δ hair/nails/energy
HEM/LYMPH	anemia / bruising / hx transfusions / blood disorder / lymphadenopathy / axillary, groin tenderness
ALLX/IMMUN	season allx / food allx / med allx / immune disorder:

SOCIAL HX	# in household ______ / lives with SP/BF/GF/SO / children ___ / tobacco Y/N #pk / sexual activity Y/N / etoh, other substances Y/N / occupation:
FAM HX	ca / HTN / MI / CAD / stroke / hyperlipidemia / DM2 / Alzheimer's / depression / osteoporosis / other:

GENERAL	well appearing / well nourished / a&o x 3 / normal mood / normal affect
NEURO	intact / abnormal **DTR:** 1 2 3 4 5 location:
SKIN + NAILS	turgor / rash / bruising / lesions // texture, distribution of hair // nails: abnormal color / nail deformity
HEAD	normocephalic / atraumatic / visible mass / palpable mass / depression / scarring
EYES	acuity intact / conjunctiva clear / EOM intact / PERRLA / fundi: normal discs and vessels / icterus / exudate / hemorrhage
EARS	EACs clear / TM translucent, mobile / landmarks abnormal / hearing diminished
NOSE	lesions / mucosal inflammation / septum, turbinates abnormal / sinus tenderness
MOUTH	mucous membranes dry / lesions / poor dentition / caries / gingival inflammation
PHARYNX	mucosa inflammation / tonsillar hypertrophy / tonsillar exudate
NECK	supple / ROM WNL / lesion / bruit / adenopathy / thyroid enlarged, tender / mass
CARDIAC	regular rate, rhythm / S1, S2 / murmur / gallop / click / rub / PMI displacement
RESP	clear to auscultation in all fields / wheezes (insp) (exp) / rales / crackles
ABDOMEN	BSx4 / tender / organomegaly / mass / hernia
RECTAL	abnormal tone / hemorrhoids (int/ext) / palpable mass
BACK	abnormal curvature / tenderness / CVAT / Δ ROM
EXTREMITIES	amputation / deformity / edema / varicosities / + pulses
MSK	abnormal gait / asymmetry / crepitation / defect / tenderness / mass / effusion / Δ ROM / instability / atrophy / abnormal strength, tone in head, neck, spine, ribs, pelvis, UE, LE / pathologic reflexes
PSYCH	A&O x3 / +recent/remote memory / insight / affect
BREAST	nipple abnormality / mass / tenderness / axillary, clavicular adenopathy
GYN/GU	lesions / d/c / uterus, adnexa tenderness / CMT // circumcised / penile lesions / urethra normal location, no d/c / testes normal / + cremasteric reflex
FEET	+ pulses / monofilament + / nails abnormal / dry, broken skin / callus

LABS	CBC / CMP / lipids / TSH / microalbumin / A1C / UA, culture / PSA / iron studies / other:

DIAGNOSTICS	XR / MRI / CT / US / cardiac / other
REFERRALS	**F/U** ___ wk ___ mo

<table>
<tr><td>Patient ID#:</td><td>Date of visit:</td></tr>
<tr><td>Reason for visit:</td><td>Age: Gender:</td></tr>
</table>

BP: **HT:**
HR: **WT:**
T: **BMI:**
O2%:   **PAIN:**

NOTES . . . .

CONST Δ appetite, energy, weight / fever / chills / sweats / fatigue
HEAD trauma / mass / tenderness / rash / lesions
EYES visionΔ / itch / d/c / tears / dry / cataracts / glaucoma / glasses, contacts
ENT hearing Δ / pain / d/c / vertigo / ? infection // epistaxis / congestion // bleeding, swelling gums / pain / sore throat / voice Δ // neck pain / lumps / swelling / difficulty swallowing

CARDIAC pain / pressure / dizzy / N / orthopnea / edema / palp / weak w exertion / hx murmurs / hx MI / HTN / HF / numb / tingle / cold extrem / slow wound healing

RESP wheeze / SOB / cough / asthma / bronch / COPD
GI abd pain / Δ in bowels / constipation / diarrhea / N V / hepatitis / gallstones / dysphagia / reflux / hemorrhoids / black, bloody stools

GU burn / pain / nocturia / polyuria / hematuria / incontinence / infection / kid. stones
GENITAL DC / sores / pain / masses / last pap ______ / sexually active Y N / dyspareunia / LMP ______ / contraception

MSK redness / swelling / warmth / pain / +/- ROM / arthritis / musc cramps / fracture / sprains / joint replacement / stiffness: AM PM

SKIN rash / pruritis / jaundice / bruising / hx skin ca / mole Δ / Δ in hair, nails / lesions / slow wound healing

BREASTS lump / pain / dc / last mammo ______ / self exams YN
NEURO HA / seizure / vertigo / memory Δ / gait Δ / speech / coord
PSYCH depression / anxiety / Δ in sleep pattern / substance, ETOH abuse / suicidal ideation / homicidal ideation

ENDO polydipsia, polyuria / heat, cold intolerance / Δ hair/nails/energy
HEM/LYMPH anemia / bruising / hx transfusions / blood disorder / lymphadenopathy / axillary, groin tenderness

ALLX/IMMUN season allx / food allx / med allx / immune disorder:

SOCIAL HX # in household ______ / lives with SP/BF/GF/SO / children __ / tobacco Y/N #pk / sexual activity Y/N / etoh, other substances Y/N / occupation:
FAM HX ca / HTN / MI / CAD / stroke / hyperlipidemia / DM2 / Alzheimer's / depression / osteoporosis / other:

GENERAL well appearing / well nourished / a&o x 3 / normal mood / normal affect
NEURO intact / abnormal   **DTR:** 1 2 3 4 5 location:
SKIN + NAILS turgor / rash / bruising / lesions // texture, distribution of hair // nails: abnormal color / nail deformity

HEAD normocephalic / atraumatic / visible mass / palpable mass / depression / scarring
EYES acuity intact / conjunctiva clear / EOM intact / PERRLA / fundi: normal discs and vessels / icterus / exudate / hemorrhage

EARS EACs clear / TM translucent, mobile / landmarks abnormal / hearing diminished
NOSE lesions / mucosal inflammation / septum, turbinates abnormal / sinus tenderness
MOUTH mucous membranes dry / lesions / poor dentition / caries / gingival inflammation
PHARYNX mucosa inflammation / tonsillar hypertrophy / tonsillar exudate
NECK supple / ROM WNL / lesion / bruit / adenopathy / thyroid enlarged, tender / mass
CARDIAC regular rate, rhythm / S1, S2 / murmur / gallop / click / rub / PMI displacement
RESP clear to auscultation in all fields / wheezes (insp) (exp) / rales / crackles
ABDOMEN BSx4 / tender / organomegaly / mass / hernia
RECTAL abnormal tone / hemorrhoids (int/ext) / palpable mass
BACK abnormal curvature / tenderness / CVAT / Δ ROM
EXTREMITIES amputation / deformity / edema / varicosities / + pulses
MSK abnormal gait / asymmetry / crepitation / defect / tenderness / mass / effusion / Δ ROM / instability / atrophy / abnormal strength, tone in head, neck, spine, ribs, pelvis, UE, LE / pathologic reflexes

PSYCH A&O x3 / +recent/remote memory / insight / affect
BREAST nipple abnormality / mass / tenderness / axillary, clavicular adenopathy
GYN/GU lesions / d/c / uterus, adnexa tenderness / CMT // circumcised / penile lesions / urethra normal location, no d/c / testes normal / + cremasteric reflex
FEET + pulses / monofilament + / nails abnormal / dry, broken skin / callus

LABS CBC / CMP / lipids / TSH / microalbumin / A1C / UA, culture / PSA / iron studies / other:

DIAGNOSTICS XR / MRI / CT / US / cardiac / other
REFERRALS **F/U** ___ wk ___ mo

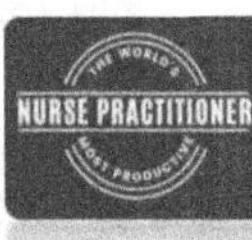

<table>
<tr><td colspan="2">
Patient ID#:
Reason for visit:
</td><td>
Date of visit:
Age: Gender:
</td></tr>
</table>

BP: **HT:**
HR: **WT:**
T: **BMI:**
O2%:   **PAIN:**

NOTES . . . .

CONST — Δ appetite, energy, weight / fever / chills / sweats / fatigue
HEAD — trauma / mass / tenderness / rash / lesions
EYES — visionΔ / itch / d/c / tears / dry / cataracts / glaucoma / glasses, contacts
ENT — hearing Δ / pain / d/c / vertigo / ? infection // epistaxis / congestion // bleeding, swelling gums / pain / sore throat / voice Δ // neck pain / lumps / swelling / difficulty swallowing

CARDIAC — pain / pressure / dizzy / N / orthopnea / edema / palp / weak w exertion / hx murmurs / hx MI / HTN / HF / numb / tingle / cold extrem / slow wound healing
RESP — wheeze / SOB / cough / asthma / bronch / COPD
GI — abd pain / Δ in bowels / constipation / diarrhea / N V / hepatitis / gallstones / dysphagia / reflux / hemorrhoids / black, bloody stools
GU — burn / pain / nocturia / polyuria / hematuria / incontinence / infection / kid. stones
GENITAL — DC / sores / pain / masses / last pap _______ / sexually active Y N / dyspareunia / LMP ________ / contraception
MSK — redness / swelling / warmth / pain / +/- ROM / arthritis / musc cramps / fracture / sprains / joint replacement / stiffness: AM PM
SKIN — rash / pruritis / jaundice / bruising / hx skin ca / mole Δ / Δ in hair, nails / lesions / slow wound healing
BREASTS — lump / pain / dc / last mammo ______ / self exams YN
NEURO — HA / seizure / vertigo / memory Δ / gait Δ / speech / coord
PSYCH — depression / anxiety / Δ in sleep pattern / substance, ETOH abuse / suicidal ideation / homicidal ideation
ENDO — polydipsia, polyuria / heat, cold intolerance / Δ hair/nails/energy
HEM/LYMPH — anemia / bruising / hx transfusions / blood disorder / lymphadenopathy / axillary, groin tenderness
ALLX/IMMUN — season allx / food allx / med allx / immune disorder:

SOCIAL HX — # in household ________ / lives with SP/BF/GF/SO / children ___ / tobacco Y/N #pk / sexual activity Y/N / etoh, other substances Y/N / occupation:
FAM HX — ca / HTN / MI / CAD / stroke / hyperlipidemia / DM2 / Alzheimer's / depression / osteoporosis / other:

GENERAL — well appearing / well nourished / a&o x 3 / normal mood / normal affect
NEURO — intact / abnormal   **DTR:** 1 2 3 4 5 location:
SKIN + NAILS — turgor / rash / bruising / lesions // texture, distribution of hair // nails: abnormal color / nail deformity
HEAD — normocephalic / atraumatic / visible mass / palpable mass / depression / scarring
EYES — acuity intact / conjunctiva clear / EOM intact / PERRLA / fundi: normal discs and vessels / icterus / exudate / hemorrhage
EARS — EACs clear / TM translucent, mobile / landmarks abnormal / hearing diminished
NOSE — lesions / mucosal inflammation / septum, turbinates abnormal / sinus tenderness
MOUTH — mucous membranes dry / lesions / poor dentition / caries / gingival inflammation
PHARYNX — mucosa inflammation / tonsillar hypertrophy / tonsillar exudate
NECK — supple / ROM WNL / lesion / bruit / adenopathy / thyroid enlarged, tender / mass
CARDIAC — regular rate, rhythm / S1, S2 / murmur / gallop / click / rub / PMI displacement
RESP — clear to auscultation in all fields / wheezes (insp) (exp) / rales / crackles
ABDOMEN — BSx4 / tender / organomegaly / mass / hernia
RECTAL — abnormal tone / hemorrhoids (int/ext) / palpable mass
BACK — abnormal curvature / tenderness / CVAT / Δ ROM
EXTREMITIES — amputation / deformity / edema / varicosities / + pulses
MSK — abnormal gait / asymmetry / crepitation / defect / tenderness / mass / effusion / Δ ROM / instability / atrophy / abnormal strength, tone in head, neck, spine, ribs, pelvis, UE, LE / pathologic reflexes
PSYCH — A&O x3 / +recent/remote memory / insight / affect
BREAST — nipple abnormality / mass / tenderness / axillary, clavicular adenopathy
GYN/GU — lesions / d/c / uterus, adnexa tenderness / CMT // circumcised / penile lesions / urethra normal location, no d/c / testes normal / + cremasteric reflex
FEET — + pulses / monofilament + / nails abnormal / dry, broken skin / callus

LABS — CBC / CMP / lipids / TSH / microalbumin / A1C / UA, culture / PSA / iron studies / other:

DIAGNOSTICS — XR / MRI / CT / US / cardiac / other
REFERRALS —   **F/U** ___ wk ___ mo

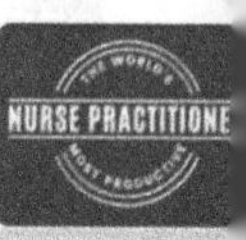

<table>
<tr><td colspan="2">

Patient ID#:   **Date of visit:**

Reason for visit: **Age:**   **Gender:**

</td><td>

BP: **HT:**

HR: **WT:**

T: **BMI:**

O2%:   **PAIN:**

</td></tr>
</table>

NOTES . . . .

CONST	Δ appetite, energy, weight / fever / chills / sweats / fatigue
HEAD	trauma / mass / tenderness / rash / lesions
EYES	visionΔ / itch / d/c / tears / dry / cataracts / glaucoma / glasses, contacts
ENT	hearing Δ / pain / d/c / vertigo / ? infection // epistaxis / congestion // bleeding, swelling gums / pain / sore throat / voice Δ // neck pain / lumps / swelling / difficulty swallowing
CARDIAC	pain / pressure / dizzy / N / orthopnea / edema / palp / weak w exertion / hx murmurs / hx MI / HTN / HF / numb / tingle / cold extrem / slow wound healing
RESP	wheeze / SOB / cough / asthma / bronch / COPD
GI	abd pain / Δ in bowels / constipation / diarrhea / N V / hepatitis / gallstones / dysphagia / reflux / hemorrhoids / black, bloody stools
GU	burn / pain / nocturia / polyuria / hematuria / incontinence / infection / kid. stones
GENITAL	DC / sores / pain / masses / last pap _____ / sexually active Y N / dyspareunia / LMP _____ / contraception
MSK	redness / swelling / warmth / pain / +/- ROM / arthritis / musc cramps / fracture / sprains / joint replacement / stiffness: AM PM
SKIN	rash / pruritis / jaundice / bruising / hx skin ca / mole Δ / Δ in hair, nails / lesions / slow wound healing
BREASTS	lump / pain / dc / last mammo _____ / self exams YN
NEURO	HA / seizure / vertigo / memory Δ / gait Δ / speech / coord
PSYCH	depression / anxiety / Δ in sleep pattern / substance, ETOH abuse / suicidal ideation / homicidal ideation
ENDO	polydipsia, polyuria / heat, cold intolerance / Δ hair/nails/energy
HEM/LYMPH	anemia / bruising / hx transfusions / blood disorder / lymphadenopathy / axillary, groin tenderness
ALLX/IMMUN	season allx / food allx / med allx / immune disorder:

SOCIAL HX	# in household _____ / lives with SP/BF/GF/SO / children __ / tobacco Y/N #pk / sexual activity Y/N / etoh, other substances Y/N / occupation:
FAM HX	ca / HTN / MI / CAD / stroke / hyperlipidemia / DM2 / Alzheimer's / depression / osteoporosis / other:

GENERAL	well appearing / well nourished / a&o x 3 / normal mood / normal affect
NEURO	intact / abnormal **DTR:** 1 2 3 4 5 location:
SKIN + NAILS	turgor / rash / bruising / lesions // texture, distribution of hair // nails: abnormal color / nail deformity
HEAD	normocephalic / atraumatic / visible mass / palpable mass / depression / scarring
EYES	acuity intact / conjunctiva clear / EOM intact / PERRLA / fundi: normal discs and vessels / icterus / exudate / hemorrhage
EARS	EACs clear / TM translucent, mobile / landmarks abnormal / hearing diminished
NOSE	lesions / mucosal inflammation / septum, turbinates abnormal / sinus tenderness
MOUTH	mucous membranes dry / lesions / poor dentition / caries / gingival inflammation
PHARYNX	mucosa inflammation / tonsillar hypertrophy / tonsillar exudate
NECK	supple / ROM WNL / lesion / bruit / adenopathy / thyroid enlarged, tender / mass
CARDIAC	regular rate, rhythm / S1, S2 / murmur / gallop / click / rub / PMI displacement
RESP	clear to auscultation in all fields / wheezes (insp) (exp) / rales / crackles
ABDOMEN	BSx4 / tender / organomegaly / mass / hernia
RECTAL	abnormal tone / hemorrhoids (int/ext) / palpable mass
BACK	abnormal curvature / tenderness / CVAT / Δ ROM
EXTREMITIES	amputation / deformity / edema / varicosities / + pulses
MSK	abnormal gait / asymmetry / crepitation / defect / tenderness / mass / effusion / Δ ROM / instability / atrophy / abnormal strength, tone in head, neck, spine, ribs, pelvis, UE, LE / pathologic reflexes
PSYCH	A&O x3 / +recent/remote memory / insight / affect
BREAST	nipple abnormality / mass / tenderness / axillary, clavicular adenopathy
GYN/GU	lesions / d/c / uterus, adnexa tenderness / CMT // circumcised / penile lesions / urethra normal location, no d/c / testes normal / + cremasteric reflex
FEET	+ pulses / monofilament + / nails abnormal / dry, broken skin / callus

LABS	CBC / CMP / lipids / TSH / microalbumin / A1C / UA, culture / PSA / iron studies / other:

DIAGNOSTICS	XR / MRI / CT / US / cardiac / other
REFERRALS	**F/U** ___ wk ___ mo

<table>
<tr><td>

Patient ID#:
Reason for visit:
</td><td>

Date of visit:
Age: Gender:
</td></tr>
</table>

BP:	**HT:**
HR:	**WT:**
T:	**BMI:**
O2%:	**PAIN:**

NOTES . . . .

CONST Δ appetite, energy, weight / fever / chills / sweats / fatigue
HEAD trauma / mass / tenderness / rash / lesions
EYES visionΔ / itch / d/c / tears / dry / cataracts / glaucoma / glasses, contacts
ENT hearing Δ / pain / d/c / vertigo / ? infection // epistaxis / congestion // bleeding, swelling gums / pain / sore throat / voice Δ // neck pain / lumps / swelling / difficulty swallowing

CARDIAC pain / pressure / dizzy / N / orthopnea / edema / palp / weak w exertion / hx murmurs / hx MI / HTN / HF / numb / tingle / cold extrem / slow wound healing
RESP wheeze / SOB / cough / asthma / bronch / COPD
GI abd pain / Δ in bowels / constipation / diarrhea / N V / hepatitis / gallstones / dysphagia / reflux / hemorrhoids / black, bloody stools
GU burn / pain / nocturia / polyuria / hematuria / incontinence / infection / kid. stones
GENITAL DC / sores / pain / masses / last pap _____ / sexually active Y N / dyspareunia / LMP   / contraception
MSK redness / swelling / warmth / pain / +/- ROM / arthritis / musc cramps / fracture / sprains / joint replacement / stiffness: AM PM
SKIN rash / pruritis / jaundice / bruising / hx skin ca / mole Δ / Δ in hair, nails / lesions / slow wound healing
BREASTS lump / pain / dc / last mammo   / self exams YN
NEURO HA / seizure / vertigo / memory Δ / gait Δ / speech / coord
PSYCH depression / anxiety / Δ in sleep pattern / substance, ETOH abuse / suicidal ideation / homicidal ideation
ENDO polydipsia, polyuria / heat, cold intolerance / Δ hair/nails/energy
HEM/LYMPH anemia / bruising / hx transfusions / blood disorder / lymphadenopathy / axillary, groin tenderness
ALLX/IMMUN season allx / food allx / med allx / immune disorder:

SOCIAL HX # in household _____ / lives with SP/BF/GF/SO / children __ / tobacco Y/N #pk / sexual activity Y/N / etoh, other substances Y/N / occupation:
FAM HX ca / HTN / MI / CAD / stroke / hyperlipidemia / DM2 / Alzheimer's / depression / osteoporosis / other:

GENERAL well appearing / well nourished / a&o x 3 / normal mood / normal affect
NEURO intact / abnormal   **DTR:** 1 2 3 4 5 location:
SKIN + NAILS turgor / rash / bruising / lesions // texture, distribution of hair // nails: abnormal color / nail deformity
HEAD normocephalic / atraumatic / visible mass / palpable mass / depression / scarring
EYES acuity intact / conjunctiva clear / EOM intact / PERRLA / fundi: normal discs and vessels / icterus / exudate / hemorrhage
EARS EACs clear / TM translucent, mobile / landmarks abnormal / hearing diminished
NOSE lesions / mucosal inflammation / septum, turbinates abnormal / sinus tenderness
MOUTH mucous membranes dry / lesions / poor dentition / caries / gingival inflammation
PHARYNX mucosa inflammation / tonsillar hypertrophy / tonsillar exudate
NECK supple / ROM WNL / lesion / bruit / adenopathy / thyroid enlarged, tender / mass
CARDIAC regular rate, rhythm / S1, S2 / murmur / gallop / click / rub / PMI displacement
RESP clear to auscultation in all fields / wheezes (insp) (exp) / rales / crackles
ABDOMEN BSx4 / tender / organomegaly / mass / hernia
RECTAL abnormal tone / hemorrhoids (int/ext) / palpable mass
BACK abnormal curvature / tenderness / CVAT / Δ ROM
EXTREMITIES amputation / deformity / edema / varicosities / + pulses
MSK abnormal gait / asymmetry / crepitation / defect / tenderness / mass / effusion / Δ ROM / instability / atrophy / abnormal strength, tone in head, neck, spine, ribs, pelvis, UE, LE / pathologic reflexes
PSYCH A&O x3 / +recent/remote memory / insight / affect
BREAST nipple abnormality / mass / tenderness / axillary, clavicular adenopathy
GYN/GU lesions / d/c / uterus, adnexa tenderness / CMT // circumcised / penile lesions / urethra normal location, no d/c / testes normal / + cremasteric reflex
FEET + pulses / monofilament + / nails abnormal / dry, broken skin / callus

LABS CBC / CMP / lipids / TSH / microalbumin / A1C / UA, culture / PSA / iron studies / other:

DIAGNOSTICS XR / MRI / CT / US / cardiac / other
REFERRALS   **F/U** ___ wk ___ mo

| Patient ID#: | Date of visit: |
| Reason for visit: | Age: Gender: |

BP: HT:
HR: WT:
T: BMI:
O2%:   PAIN:

NOTES . . . .

CONST	Δ appetite, energy, weight / fever / chills / sweats / fatigue
HEAD	trauma / mass / tenderness / rash / lesions
EYES	visionΔ / itch / d/c / tears / dry / cataracts / glaucoma / glasses, contacts
ENT	hearing Δ / pain / d/c / vertigo / ? infection // epistaxis / congestion // bleeding, swelling gums / pain / sore throat / voice Δ // neck pain / lumps / swelling / difficulty swallowing
CARDIAC	pain / pressure / dizzy / N / orthopnea / edema / palp / weak w exertion / hx murmurs / hx MI / HTN / HF / numb / tingle / cold extrem / slow wound healing
RESP	wheeze / SOB / cough / asthma / bronch / COPD
GI	abd pain / Δ in bowels / constipation / diarrhea / N V / hepatitis / gallstones / dysphagia / reflux / hemorrhoids / black, bloody stools
GU	burn / pain / nocturia / polyuria / hematuria / incontinence / infection / kid. stones
GENITAL	DC / sores / pain / masses / last pap _____ / sexually active Y N / dyspareunia / LMP / contraception
MSK	redness / swelling / warmth / pain / +/- ROM / arthritis / musc cramps / fracture / sprains / joint replacement / stiffness: AM PM
SKIN	rash / pruritis / jaundice / bruising / hx skin ca / mole Δ / Δ in hair, nails / lesions / slow wound healing
BREASTS	lump / pain / dc / last mammo / self exams YN
NEURO	HA / seizure / vertigo / memory Δ / gait Δ / speech / coord
PSYCH	depression / anxiety / Δ in sleep pattern / substance, ETOH abuse / suicidal ideation / homicidal ideation
ENDO	polydipsia, polyuria / heat, cold intolerance / Δ hair/nails/energy
HEM/LYMPH	anemia / bruising / hx transfusions / blood disorder / lymphadenopathy / axillary, groin tenderness
ALLX/IMMUN	season allx / food allx / med allx / immune disorder:
SOCIAL HX	# in household _____ / lives with SP/BF/GF/SO / children __ / tobacco Y/N #pk / sexual activity Y/N / etoh, other substances Y/N / occupation:
FAM HX	ca / HTN / MI / CAD / stroke / hyperlipidemia / DM2 / Alzheimer's / depression / osteoporosis / other:
GENERAL	well appearing / well nourished / a&o x 3 / normal mood / normal affect
NEURO	intact / abnormal **DTR:** 1 2 3 4 5 location:
SKIN + NAILS	turgor / rash / bruising / lesions // texture, distribution of hair // nails: abnormal color / nail deformity
HEAD	normocephalic / atraumatic / visible mass / palpable mass / depression / scarring
EYES	acuity intact / conjunctiva clear / EOM intact / PERRLA / fundi: normal discs and vessels / icterus / exudate / hemorrhage
EARS	EACs clear / TM translucent, mobile / landmarks abnormal / hearing diminished
NOSE	lesions / mucosal inflammation / septum, turbinates abnormal / sinus tenderness
MOUTH	mucous membranes dry / lesions / poor dentition / caries / gingival inflammation
PHARYNX	mucosa inflammation / tonsillar hypertrophy / tonsillar exudate
NECK	supple / ROM WNL / lesion / bruit / adenopathy / thyroid enlarged, tender / mass
CARDIAC	regular rate, rhythm / S1, S2 / murmur / gallop / click / rub / PMI displacement
RESP	clear to auscultation in all fields / wheezes (insp) (exp) / rales / crackles
ABDOMEN	BSx4 / tender / organomegaly / mass / hernia
RECTAL	abnormal tone / hemorrhoids (int/ext) / palpable mass
BACK	abnormal curvature / tenderness / CVAT / Δ ROM
EXTREMITIES	amputation / deformity / edema / varicosities / + pulses
MSK	abnormal gait / asymmetry / crepitation / defect / tenderness / mass / effusion / Δ ROM / instability / atrophy / abnormal strength, tone in head, neck, spine, ribs, pelvis, UE, LE / pathologic reflexes
PSYCH	A&O x3 / +recent/remote memory / insight / affect
BREAST	nipple abnormality / mass / tenderness / axillary, clavicular adenopathy
GYN/GU	lesions / d/c / uterus, adnexa tenderness / CMT // circumcised / penile lesions / urethra normal location, no d/c / testes normal / + cremasteric reflex
FEET	+ pulses / monofilament + / nails abnormal / dry, broken skin / callus
LABS	CBC / CMP / lipids / TSH / microalbumin / A1C / UA, culture / PSA / iron studies / other:
DIAGNOSTICS	XR / MRI / CT / US / cardiac / other
REFERRALS	**F/U** ___ wk ___ mo

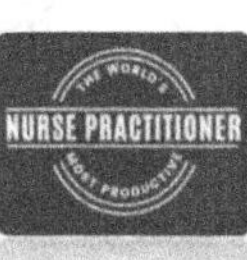

<table>
<tr><td>Patient ID#:
Reason for visit:</td><td>Date of visit:
Age: Gender:</td></tr>
</table>

BP: HT:
HR: WT:
T: BMI:
O2%:   PAIN:

NOTES . . . .

CONST Δ appetite, energy, weight / fever / chills / sweats / fatigue
HEAD trauma / mass / tenderness / rash / lesions
EYES visionΔ / itch / d/c / tears / dry / cataracts / glaucoma / glasses, contacts
ENT hearing Δ / pain / d/c / vertigo / ? infection // epistaxis / congestion // bleeding, swelling gums / pain / sore throat / voice Δ // neck pain / lumps / swelling / difficulty swallowing

CARDIAC pain / pressure / dizzy / N / orthopnea / edema / palp / weak w exertion / hx murmurs / hx MI / HTN / HF / numb / tingle / cold extrem / slow wound healing
RESP wheeze / SOB / cough / asthma / bronch / COPD
GI abd pain / Δ in bowels / constipation / diarrhea / N V / hepatitis / gallstones / dysphagia / reflux / hemorrhoids / black, bloody stools
GU burn / pain / nocturia / polyuria / hematuria / incontinence / infection / kid. stones
GENITAL DC / sores / pain / masses / last pap ______ / sexually active Y N / dyspareunia / LMP ______ / contraception
MSK redness / swelling / warmth / pain / +/- ROM / arthritis / musc cramps / fracture / sprains / joint replacement / stiffness: AM PM
SKIN rash / pruritis / jaundice / bruising / hx skin ca / mole Δ / Δ in hair, nails / lesions / slow wound healing
BREASTS lump / pain / dc / last mammo ______ / self exams YN
NEURO HA / seizure / vertigo / memory Δ / gait Δ / speech / coord
PSYCH depression / anxiety / Δ in sleep pattern / substance, ETOH abuse / suicidal ideation / homicidal ideation
ENDO polydipsia, polyuria / heat, cold intolerance / Δ hair/nails/energy
HEM/LYMPH anemia / bruising / hx transfusions / blood disorder / lymphadenopathy / axillary, groin tenderness
ALLX/IMMUN season allx / food allx / med allx / immune disorder:

SOCIAL HX # in household ______ / lives with SP/BF/GF/SO / children __ / tobacco Y/N #pk / sexual activity Y/N / etoh, other substances Y/N / occupation:
FAM HX ca / HTN / MI / CAD / stroke / hyperlipidemia / DM2 / Alzheimer's / depression / osteoporosis / other:

GENERAL well appearing / well nourished / a&o x 3 / normal mood / normal affect
NEURO intact / abnormal   **DTR:** 1 2 3 4 5 location:
SKIN + NAILS turgor / rash / bruising / lesions // texture, distribution of hair // nails: abnormal color / nail deformity
HEAD normocephalic / atraumatic / visible mass / palpable mass / depression / scarring
EYES acuity intact / conjunctiva clear / EOM intact / PERRLA / fundi: normal discs and vessels / icterus / exudate / hemorrhage
EARS EACs clear / TM translucent, mobile / landmarks abnormal / hearing diminished
NOSE lesions / mucosal inflammation / septum, turbinates abnormal / sinus tenderness
MOUTH mucous membranes dry / lesions / poor dentition / caries / gingival inflammation
PHARYNX mucosa inflammation / tonsillar hypertrophy / tonsillar exudate
NECK supple / ROM WNL / lesion / bruit / adenopathy / thyroid enlarged, tender / mass
CARDIAC regular rate, rhythm / S1, S2 / murmur / gallop / click / rub / PMI displacement
RESP clear to auscultation in all fields / wheezes (insp) (exp) / rales / crackles
ABDOMEN BSx4 / tender / organomegaly / mass / hernia
RECTAL abnormal tone / hemorrhoids (int/ext) / palpable mass
BACK abnormal curvature / tenderness / CVAT / Δ ROM
EXTREMITIES amputation / deformity / edema / varicosities / + pulses
MSK abnormal gait / asymmetry / crepitation / defect / tenderness / mass / effusion / Δ ROM / instability / atrophy / abnormal strength, tone in head, neck, spine, ribs, pelvis, UE, LE / pathologic reflexes
PSYCH A&O x3 / +recent/remote memory / insight / affect
BREAST nipple abnormality / mass / tenderness / axillary, clavicular adenopathy
GYN/GU lesions / d/c / uterus, adnexa tenderness / CMT // circumcised / penile lesions / urethra normal location, no d/c / testes normal / + cremasteric reflex
FEET + pulses / monofilament + / nails abnormal / dry, broken skin / callus

LABS CBC / CMP / lipids / TSH / microalbumin / A1C / UA, culture / PSA / iron studies / other:

DIAGNOSTICS XR / MRI / CT / US / cardiac / other
REFERRALS   **F/U** ___ wk ___ mo

<table>
<tr><td colspan="2">
Patient ID#:
Reason for visit:
</td><td>
Date of visit:
Age: Gender:
</td></tr>
</table>

<table>
<tr><td>BP:</td><td>HT:</td></tr>
<tr><td>HR:</td><td>WT:</td></tr>
<tr><td>T:</td><td>BMI:</td></tr>
<tr><td>O2%:</td><td>PAIN:</td></tr>
</table>

NOTES . . . .

CONST	Δ appetite, energy, weight / fever / chills / sweats / fatigue
HEAD	trauma / mass / tenderness / rash / lesions
EYES	visionΔ / itch / d/c / tears / dry / cataracts / glaucoma / glasses, contacts
ENT	hearing Δ / pain / d/c / vertigo / ? infection // epistaxis / congestion // bleeding, swelling gums / pain / sore throat / voice Δ // neck pain / lumps / swelling / difficulty swallowing
CARDIAC	pain / pressure / dizzy / N / orthopnea / edema / palp / weak w exertion / hx murmurs / hx MI / HTN / HF / numb / tingle / cold extrem / slow wound healing
RESP	wheeze / SOB / cough / asthma / bronch / COPD
GI	abd pain / Δ in bowels / constipation / diarrhea / N V / hepatitis / gallstones / dysphagia / reflux / hemorrhoids / black, bloody stools
GU	burn / pain / nocturia / polyuria / hematuria / incontinence / infection / kid. stones
GENITAL	DC / sores / pain / masses / last pap ______ / sexually active Y N / dyspareunia / LMP ______ / contraception
MSK	redness / swelling / warmth / pain / +/- ROM / arthritis / musc cramps / fracture / sprains / joint replacement / stiffness: AM PM
SKIN	rash / pruritis / jaundice / bruising / hx skin ca / mole Δ / Δ in hair, nails / lesions / slow wound healing
BREASTS	lump / pain / dc / last mammo ______ / self exams YN
NEURO	HA / seizure / vertigo / memory Δ / gait Δ / speech / coord
PSYCH	depression / anxiety / Δ in sleep pattern / substance, ETOH abuse / suicidal ideation / homicidal ideation
ENDO	polydipsia, polyuria / heat, cold intolerance / Δ hair/nails/energy
HEM/LYMPH	anemia / bruising / hx transfusions / blood disorder / lymphadenopathy / axillary, groin tenderness
ALLX/IMMUN	season allx / food allx / med allx / immune disorder:

SOCIAL HX	# in household ______ / lives with SP/BF/GF/SO / children __ / tobacco Y/N #pk / sexual activity Y/N / etoh, other substances Y/N / occupation:
FAM HX	ca / HTN / MI / CAD / stroke / hyperlipidemia / DM2 / Alzheimer's / depression / osteoporosis / other:

GENERAL	well appearing / well nourished / a&o x 3 / normal mood / normal affect
NEURO	intact / abnormal **DTR:** 1 2 3 4 5 location:
SKIN + NAILS	turgor / rash / bruising / lesions // texture, distribution of hair // nails: abnormal color / nail deformity
HEAD	normocephalic / atraumatic / visible mass / palpable mass / depression / scarring
EYES	acuity intact / conjunctiva clear / EOM intact / PERRLA / fundi: normal discs and vessels / icterus / exudate / hemorrhage
EARS	EACs clear / TM translucent, mobile / landmarks abnormal / hearing diminished
NOSE	lesions / mucosal inflammation / septum, turbinates abnormal / sinus tenderness
MOUTH	mucous membranes dry / lesions / poor dentition / caries / gingival inflammation
PHARYNX	mucosa inflammation / tonsillar hypertrophy / tonsillar exudate
NECK	supple / ROM WNL / lesion / bruit / adenopathy / thyroid enlarged, tender / mass
CARDIAC	regular rate, rhythm / S1, S2 / murmur / gallop / click / rub / PMI displacement
RESP	clear to auscultation in all fields / wheezes (insp) (exp) / rales / crackles
ABDOMEN	BSx4 / tender / organomegaly / mass / hernia
RECTAL	abnormal tone / hemorrhoids (int/ext) / palpable mass
BACK	abnormal curvature / tenderness / CVAT / Δ ROM
EXTREMITIES	amputation / deformity / edema / varicosities / + pulses
MSK	abnormal gait / asymmetry / crepitation / defect / tenderness / mass / effusion / Δ ROM / instability / atrophy / abnormal strength, tone in head, neck, spine, ribs, pelvis, UE, LE / pathologic reflexes
PSYCH	A&O x3 / +recent/remote memory / insight / affect
BREAST	nipple abnormality / mass / tenderness / axillary, clavicular adenopathy
GYN/GU	lesions / d/c / uterus, adnexa tenderness / CMT // circumcised / penile lesions / urethra normal location, no d/c / testes normal / + cremasteric reflex
FEET	+ pulses / monofilament + / nails abnormal / dry, broken skin / callus

LABS	CBC / CMP / lipids / TSH / microalbumin / A1C / UA, culture / PSA / iron studies / other:

DIAGNOSTICS	XR / MRI / CT / US / cardiac / other
REFERRALS	**F/U** ___ wk ___ mo

<table>
<tr><td colspan="2">

Patient ID#:

Reason for visit:

</td><td>

Date of visit:

Age: **Gender:**

</td></tr>
</table>

BP:	HT:
HR:	WT:
T:	BMI:
O2%:	PAIN:

NOTES . . . .

CONST	Δ appetite, energy, weight / fever / chills / sweats / fatigue
HEAD	trauma / mass / tenderness / rash / lesions
EYES	visionΔ / itch / d/c / tears / dry / cataracts / glaucoma / glasses, contacts
ENT	hearing Δ / pain / d/c / vertigo / ? infection // epistaxis / congestion // bleeding, swelling gums / pain / sore throat / voice Δ // neck pain / lumps / swelling / difficulty swallowing
CARDIAC	pain / pressure / dizzy / N / orthopnea / edema / palp / weak w exertion / hx murmurs / hx MI / HTN / HF / numb / tingle / cold extrem / slow wound healing
RESP	wheeze / SOB / cough / asthma / bronch / COPD
GI	abd pain / Δ in bowels / constipation / diarrhea / N V / hepatitis / gallstones / dysphagia / reflux / hemorrhoids / black, bloody stools
GU	burn / pain / nocturia / polyuria / hematuria / incontinence / infection / kid. stones
GENITAL	DC / sores / pain / masses / last pap ______ / sexually active Y N / dyspareunia / LMP ______ / contraception
MSK	redness / swelling / warmth / pain / +/- ROM / arthritis / musc cramps / fracture / sprains / joint replacement / stiffness: AM PM
SKIN	rash / pruritis / jaundice / bruising / hx skin ca / mole Δ / Δ in hair, nails / lesions / slow wound healing
BREASTS	lump / pain / dc / last mammo ______ / self exams YN
NEURO	HA / seizure / vertigo / memory Δ / gait Δ / speech / coord
PSYCH	depression / anxiety / Δ in sleep pattern / substance, ETOH abuse / suicidal ideation / homicidal ideation
ENDO	polydipsia, polyuria / heat, cold intolerance / Δ hair/nails/energy
HEM/LYMPH	anemia / bruising / hx transfusions / blood disorder / lymphadenopathy / axillary, groin tenderness
ALLX/IMMUN	season allx / food allx / med allx / immune disorder:

SOCIAL HX	# in household ______ / lives with SP/BF/GF/SO / children __ / tobacco Y/N #pk / sexual activity Y/N / etoh, other substances Y/N / occupation:
FAM HX	ca / HTN / MI / CAD / stroke / hyperlipidemia / DM2 / Alzheimer's / depression / osteoporosis / other:

GENERAL	well appearing / well nourished / a&o x 3 / normal mood / normal affect
NEURO	intact / abnormal **DTR:** 1 2 3 4 5 location:
SKIN + NAILS	turgor / rash / bruising / lesions // texture, distribution of hair // nails: abnormal color / nail deformity
HEAD	normocephalic / atraumatic / visible mass / palpable mass / depression / scarring
EYES	acuity intact / conjunctiva clear / EOM intact / PERRLA / fundi: normal discs and vessels / icterus / exudate / hemorrhage
EARS	EACs clear / TM translucent, mobile / landmarks abnormal / hearing diminished
NOSE	lesions / mucosal inflammation / septum, turbinates abnormal / sinus tenderness
MOUTH	mucous membranes dry / lesions / poor dentition / caries / gingival inflammation
PHARYNX	mucosa inflammation / tonsillar hypertrophy / tonsillar exudate
NECK	supple / ROM WNL / lesion / bruit / adenopathy / thyroid enlarged, tender / mass
CARDIAC	regular rate, rhythm / S1, S2 / murmur / gallop / click / rub / PMI displacement
RESP	clear to auscultation in all fields / wheezes (insp) (exp) / rales / crackles
ABDOMEN	BSx4 / tender / organomegaly / mass / hernia
RECTAL	abnormal tone / hemorrhoids (int/ext) / palpable mass
BACK	abnormal curvature / tenderness / CVAT / Δ ROM
EXTREMITIES	amputation / deformity / edema / varicosities / + pulses
MSK	abnormal gait / asymmetry / crepitation / defect / tenderness / mass / effusion / Δ ROM / instability / atrophy / abnormal strength, tone in head, neck, spine, ribs, pelvis, UE, LE / pathologic reflexes
PSYCH	A&O x3 / +recent/remote memory / insight / affect
BREAST	nipple abnormality / mass / tenderness / axillary, clavicular adenopathy
GYN/GU	lesions / d/c / uterus, adnexa tenderness / CMT // circumcised / penile lesions / urethra normal location, no d/c / testes normal / + cremasteric reflex
FEET	+ pulses / monofilament + / nails abnormal / dry, broken skin / callus

LABS	CBC / CMP / lipids / TSH / microalbumin / A1C / UA, culture / PSA / iron studies / other:

DIAGNOSTICS	XR / MRI / CT / US / cardiac / other
REFERRALS	**F/U** ___ wk ___ mo

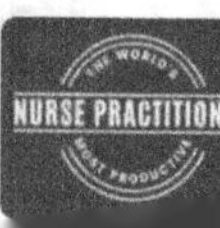

| Patient ID#: | Date of visit: |
| Reason for visit: | Age: Gender: |

BP: HT:
HR: WT:
T: BMI:
O2%: PAIN:

NOTES . . . .

CONST	Δ appetite, energy, weight / fever / chills / sweats / fatigue
HEAD	trauma / mass / tenderness / rash / lesions
EYES	visionΔ / itch / d/c / tears / dry / cataracts / glaucoma / glasses, contacts
ENT	hearing Δ / pain / d/c / vertigo / ? infection // epistaxis / congestion // bleeding, swelling gums / pain / sore throat / voice Δ // neck pain / lumps / swelling / difficulty swallowing
CARDIAC	pain / pressure / dizzy / N / orthopnea / edema / palp / weak w exertion / hx murmurs / hx MI / HTN / HF / numb / tingle / cold extrem / slow wound healing
RESP	wheeze / SOB / cough / asthma / bronch / COPD
GI	abd pain / Δ in bowels / constipation / diarrhea / N V / hepatitis / gallstones / dysphagia / reflux / hemorrhoids / black, bloody stools
GU	burn / pain / nocturia / polyuria / hematuria / incontinence / infection / kid. stones
GENITAL	DC / sores / pain / masses / last pap ______ / sexually active Y N / dyspareunia / LMP ______ / contraception
MSK	redness / swelling / warmth / pain / +/- ROM / arthritis / musc cramps / fracture / sprains / joint replacement / stiffness: AM PM
SKIN	rash / pruritis / jaundice / bruising / hx skin ca / mole Δ / Δ in hair, nails / lesions / slow wound healing
BREASTS	lump / pain / dc / last mammo ______ / self exams YN
NEURO	HA / seizure / vertigo / memory Δ / gait Δ / speech / coord
PSYCH	depression / anxiety / Δ in sleep pattern / substance, ETOH abuse / suicidal ideation / homicidal ideation
ENDO	polydipsia, polyuria / heat, cold intolerance / Δ hair/nails/energy
HEM/LYMPH	anemia / bruising / hx transfusions / blood disorder / lymphadenopathy / axillary, groin tenderness
ALLX/IMMUN	season allx / food allx / med allx / immune disorder:

| **SOCIAL HX** | # in household ______ / lives with SP/BF/GF/SO / children __ / tobacco Y/N #pk / sexual activity Y/N / etoh, other substances Y/N / occupation: |
| **FAM HX** | ca / HTN / MI / CAD / stroke / hyperlipidemia / DM2 / Alzheimer's / depression / osteoporosis / other: |

GENERAL	well appearing / well nourished / a&o x 3 / normal mood / normal affect
NEURO	intact / abnormal **DTR:** 1 2 3 4 5 location:
SKIN + NAILS	turgor / rash / bruising / lesions // texture, distribution of hair // nails: abnormal color / nail deformity
HEAD	normocephalic / atraumatic / visible mass / palpable mass / depression / scarring
EYES	acuity intact / conjunctiva clear / EOM intact / PERRLA / fundi: normal discs and vessels / icterus / exudate / hemorrhage
EARS	EACs clear / TM translucent, mobile / landmarks abnormal / hearing diminished
NOSE	lesions / mucosal inflammation / septum, turbinates abnormal / sinus tenderness
MOUTH	mucous membranes dry / lesions / poor dentition / caries / gingival inflammation
PHARYNX	mucosa inflammation / tonsillar hypertrophy / tonsillar exudate
NECK	supple / ROM WNL / lesion / bruit / adenopathy / thyroid enlarged, tender / mass
CARDIAC	regular rate, rhythm / S1, S2 / murmur / gallop / click / rub / PMI displacement
RESP	clear to auscultation in all fields / wheezes (insp) (exp) / rales / crackles
ABDOMEN	BSx4 / tender / organomegaly / mass / hernia
RECTAL	abnormal tone / hemorrhoids (int/ext) / palpable mass
BACK	abnormal curvature / tenderness / CVAT / Δ ROM
EXTREMITIES	amputation / deformity / edema / varicosities / + pulses
MSK	abnormal gait / asymmetry / crepitation / defect / tenderness / mass / effusion / Δ ROM / instability / atrophy / abnormal strength, tone in head, neck, spine, ribs, pelvis, UE, LE / pathologic reflexes
PSYCH	A&O x3 / +recent/remote memory / insight / affect
BREAST	nipple abnormality / mass / tenderness / axillary, clavicular adenopathy
GYN/GU	lesions / d/c / uterus, adnexa tenderness / CMT // circumcised / penile lesions / urethra normal location, no d/c / testes normal / + cremasteric reflex
FEET	+ pulses / monofilament + / nails abnormal / dry, broken skin / callus

| **LABS** | CBC / CMP / lipids / TSH / microalbumin / A1C / UA, culture / PSA / iron studies / other: |

| **DIAGNOSTICS** | XR / MRI / CT / US / cardiac / other |
| **REFERRALS** | **F/U** ___ wk ___ mo |

<table>
<tr><td>

Patient ID#:

Reason for visit:

</td><td>

Date of visit:

Age: **Gender:**

</td></tr>
</table>

BP: HT:
HR: WT:
T: BMI:
O2%:   PAIN:

NOTES . . . .

CONST	Δ appetite, energy, weight / fever / chills / sweats / fatigue
HEAD	trauma / mass / tenderness / rash / lesions
EYES	visionΔ / itch / d/c / tears / dry / cataracts / glaucoma / glasses, contacts
ENT	hearing Δ / pain / d/c / vertigo / ? infection // epistaxis / congestion // bleeding, swelling gums / pain / sore throat / voice Δ // neck pain / lumps / swelling / difficulty swallowing
CARDIAC	pain / pressure / dizzy / N / orthopnea / edema / palp / weak w exertion / hx murmurs / hx MI / HTN / HF / numb / tingle / cold extrem / slow wound healing
RESP	wheeze / SOB / cough / asthma / bronch / COPD
GI	abd pain / Δ in bowels / constipation / diarrhea / N V / hepatitis / gallstones / dysphagia / reflux / hemorrhoids / black, bloody stools
GU	burn / pain / nocturia / polyuria / hematuria / incontinence / infection / kid. stones
GENITAL	DC / sores / pain / masses / last pap ______ / sexually active Y N / dyspareunia / LMP ______ / contraception
MSK	redness / swelling / warmth / pain / +/- ROM / arthritis / musc cramps / fracture / sprains / joint replacement / stiffness: AM PM
SKIN	rash / pruritis / jaundice / bruising / hx skin ca / mole Δ / Δ in hair, nails / lesions / slow wound healing
BREASTS	lump / pain / dc / last mammo ______ / self exams YN
NEURO	HA / seizure / vertigo / memory Δ / gait Δ / speech / coord
PSYCH	depression / anxiety / Δ in sleep pattern / substance, ETOH abuse / suicidal ideation / homicidal ideation
ENDO	polydipsia, polyuria / heat, cold intolerance / Δ hair/nails/energy
HEM/LYMPH	anemia / bruising / hx transfusions / blood disorder / lymphadenopathy / axillary, groin tenderness
ALLX/IMMUN	season allx / food allx / med allx / immune disorder:

SOCIAL HX	# in household ______ / lives with SP/BF/GF/SO / children __ / tobacco Y/N #pk / sexual activity Y/N / etoh, other substances Y/N / occupation:
FAM HX	ca / HTN / MI / CAD / stroke / hyperlipidemia / DM2 / Alzheimer's / depression / osteoporosis / other:

GENERAL	well appearing / well nourished / a&o x 3 / normal mood / normal affect
NEURO	intact / abnormal **DTR:** 1 2 3 4 5 location:
SKIN + NAILS	turgor / rash / bruising / lesions // texture, distribution of hair // nails: abnormal color / nail deformity
HEAD	normocephalic / atraumatic / visible mass / palpable mass / depression / scarring
EYES	acuity intact / conjunctiva clear / EOM intact / PERRLA / fundi: normal discs and vessels / icterus / exudate / hemorrhage
EARS	EACs clear / TM translucent, mobile / landmarks abnormal / hearing diminished
NOSE	lesions / mucosal inflammation / septum, turbinates abnormal / sinus tenderness
MOUTH	mucous membranes dry / lesions / poor dentition / caries / gingival inflammation
PHARYNX	mucosa inflammation / tonsillar hypertrophy / tonsillar exudate
NECK	supple / ROM WNL / lesion / bruit / adenopathy / thyroid enlarged, tender / mass
CARDIAC	regular rate, rhythm / S1, S2 / murmur / gallop / click / rub / PMI displacement
RESP	clear to auscultation in all fields / wheezes (insp) (exp) / rales / crackles
ABDOMEN	BSx4 / tender / organomegaly / mass / hernia
RECTAL	abnormal tone / hemorrhoids (int/ext) / palpable mass
BACK	abnormal curvature / tenderness / CVAT / Δ ROM
EXTREMITIES	amputation / deformity / edema / varicosities / + pulses
MSK	abnormal gait / asymmetry / crepitation / defect / tenderness / mass / effusion / Δ ROM / instability / atrophy / abnormal strength, tone in head, neck, spine, ribs, pelvis, UE, LE / pathologic reflexes
PSYCH	A&O x3 / +recent/remote memory / insight / affect
BREAST	nipple abnormality / mass / tenderness / axillary, clavicular adenopathy
GYN/GU	lesions / d/c / uterus, adnexa tenderness / CMT // circumcised / penile lesions / urethra normal location, no d/c / testes normal / + cremasteric reflex
FEET	+ pulses / monofilament + / nails abnormal / dry, broken skin / callus

LABS	CBC / CMP / lipids / TSH / microalbumin / A1C / UA, culture / PSA / iron studies / other:

DIAGNOSTICS	XR / MRI / CT / US / cardiac / other
REFERRALS	**F/U** ___ wk ___ mo

<table>
<tr><td colspan="2">

Patient ID#:   **Date of visit:**
Reason for visit: **Age:**   **Gender:**

</td></tr>
</table>

BP: **HT:**
HR: **WT:**
T: **BMI:**
O2%:   **PAIN:**

NOTES . . . .

CONST	Δ appetite, energy, weight / fever / chills / sweats / fatigue
HEAD	trauma / mass / tenderness / rash / lesions
EYES	visionΔ / itch / d/c / tears / dry / cataracts / glaucoma / glasses, contacts
ENT	hearing Δ / pain / d/c / vertigo / ? infection // epistaxis / congestion // bleeding, swelling gums / pain / sore throat / voice Δ // neck pain / lumps / swelling / difficulty swallowing
CARDIAC	pain / pressure / dizzy / N / orthopnea / edema / palp / weak w exertion / hx murmurs / hx MI / HTN / HF / numb / tingle / cold extrem / slow wound healing
RESP	wheeze / SOB / cough / asthma / bronch / COPD
GI	abd pain / Δ in bowels / constipation / diarrhea / N V / hepatitis / gallstones / dysphagia / reflux / hemorrhoids / black, bloody stools
GU	burn / pain / nocturia / polyuria / hematuria / incontinence / infection / kid. stones
GENITAL	DC / sores / pain / masses / last pap ______ / sexually active Y N / dyspareunia / LMP ______ / contraception
MSK	redness / swelling / warmth / pain / +/- ROM / arthritis / musc cramps / fracture / sprains / joint replacement / stiffness: AM PM
SKIN	rash / pruritis / jaundice / bruising / hx skin ca / mole Δ / Δ in hair, nails / lesions / slow wound healing
BREASTS	lump / pain / dc / last mammo ______ / self exams YN
NEURO	HA / seizure / vertigo / memory Δ / gait Δ / speech / coord
PSYCH	depression / anxiety / Δ in sleep pattern / substance, ETOH abuse / suicidal ideation / homicidal ideation
ENDO	polydipsia, polyuria / heat, cold intolerance / Δ hair/nails/energy
HEM/LYMPH	anemia / bruising / hx transfusions / blood disorder / lymphadenopathy / axillary, groin tenderness
ALLX/IMMUN	season allx / food allx / med allx / immune disorder:

SOCIAL HX	# in household ______ / lives with SP/BF/GF/SO / children __ / tobacco Y/N #pk / sexual activity Y/N / etoh, other substances Y/N / occupation:
FAM HX	ca / HTN / MI / CAD / stroke / hyperlipidemia / DM2 / Alzheimer's / depression / osteoporosis / other:

GENERAL	well appearing / well nourished / a&o x 3 / normal mood / normal affect
NEURO	intact / abnormal **DTR:** 1 2 3 4 5 location:
SKIN + NAILS	turgor / rash / bruising / lesions // texture, distribution of hair // nails: abnormal color / nail deformity
HEAD	normocephalic / atraumatic / visible mass / palpable mass / depression / scarring
EYES	acuity intact / conjunctiva clear / EOM intact / PERRLA / fundi: normal discs and vessels / icterus / exudate / hemorrhage
EARS	EACs clear / TM translucent, mobile / landmarks abnormal / hearing diminished
NOSE	lesions / mucosal inflammation / septum, turbinates abnormal / sinus tenderness
MOUTH	mucous membranes dry / lesions / poor dentition / caries / gingival inflammation
PHARYNX	mucosa inflammation / tonsillar hypertrophy / tonsillar exudate
NECK	supple / ROM WNL / lesion / bruit / adenopathy / thyroid enlarged, tender / mass
CARDIAC	regular rate, rhythm / S1, S2 / murmur / gallop / click / rub / PMI displacement
RESP	clear to auscultation in all fields / wheezes (insp) (exp) / rales / crackles
ABDOMEN	BSx4 / tender / organomegaly / mass / hernia
RECTAL	abnormal tone / hemorrhoids (int/ext) / palpable mass
BACK	abnormal curvature / tenderness / CVAT / Δ ROM
EXTREMITIES	amputation / deformity / edema / varicosities / + pulses
MSK	abnormal gait / asymmetry / crepitation / defect / tenderness / mass / effusion / Δ ROM / instability / atrophy / abnormal strength, tone in head, neck, spine, ribs, pelvis, UE, LE / pathologic reflexes
PSYCH	A&O x3 / +recent/remote memory / insight / affect
BREAST	nipple abnormality / mass / tenderness / axillary, clavicular adenopathy
GYN/GU	lesions / d/c / uterus, adnexa tenderness / CMT // circumcised / penile lesions / urethra normal location, no d/c / testes normal / + cremasteric reflex
FEET	+ pulses / monofilament + / nails abnormal / dry, broken skin / callus

LABS	CBC / CMP / lipids / TSH / microalbumin / A1C / UA, culture / PSA / iron studies / other:

DIAGNOSTICS	XR / MRI / CT / US / cardiac / other
REFERRALS	**F/U** ___ wk ___ mo

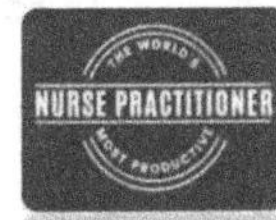

<table>
<tr><td>

Patient ID#:
Reason for visit:

</td><td>

Date of visit:
Age: Gender:

</td></tr>
</table>

BP: **HT:**
HR: **WT:**
T: **BMI:**
O2%:   **PAIN:**

NOTES . . . .

CONST Δ appetite, energy, weight / fever / chills / sweats / fatigue
HEAD trauma / mass / tenderness / rash / lesions
EYES visionΔ / itch / d/c / tears / dry / cataracts / glaucoma / glasses, contacts
ENT hearing Δ / pain / d/c / vertigo / ? infection // epistaxis / congestion // bleeding, swelling gums / pain / sore throat / voice Δ // neck pain / lumps / swelling / difficulty swallowing

CARDIAC pain / pressure / dizzy / N / orthopnea / edema / palp / weak w exertion / hx murmurs / hx MI / HTN / HF / numb / tingle / cold extrem / slow wound healing

RESP wheeze / SOB / cough / asthma / bronch / COPD
GI abd pain / Δ in bowels / constipation / diarrhea / N V / hepatitis / gallstones / dysphagia / reflux / hemorrhoids / black, bloody stools

GU burn / pain / nocturia / polyuria / hematuria / incontinence / infection / kid. stones
GENITAL DC / sores / pain / masses / last pap _____ / sexually active Y N / dyspareunia / LMP   / contraception

MSK redness / swelling / warmth / pain / +/- ROM / arthritis / musc cramps / fracture / sprains / joint replacement / stiffness: AM PM

SKIN rash / pruritis / jaundice / bruising / hx skin ca / mole Δ / Δ in hair, nails / lesions / slow wound healing

BREASTS lump / pain / dc / last mammo   / self exams YN
NEURO HA / seizure / vertigo / memory Δ / gait Δ / speech / coord
PSYCH depression / anxiety / Δ in sleep pattern / substance, ETOH abuse / suicidal ideation / homicidal ideation

ENDO polydipsia, polyuria / heat, cold intolerance / Δ hair/nails/energy
HEM/LYMPH anemia / bruising / hx transfusions / blood disorder / lymphadenopathy / axillary, groin tenderness

ALLX/IMMUN season allx / food allx / med allx / immune disorder:

SOCIAL HX # in household _____ / lives with SP/BF/GF/SO / children __ / tobacco Y/N #pk / sexual activity Y/N / etoh, other substances Y/N / occupation:
FAM HX ca / HTN / MI / CAD / stroke / hyperlipidemia / DM2 / Alzheimer's / depression / osteoporosis / other:

GENERAL well appearing / well nourished / a&o x 3 / normal mood / normal affect
NEURO intact / abnormal   **DTR:** 1 2 3 4 5 location:
SKIN + NAILS turgor / rash / bruising / lesions // texture, distribution of hair // nails: abnormal color / nail deformity

HEAD normocephalic / atraumatic / visible mass / palpable mass / depression / scarring
EYES acuity intact / conjunctiva clear / EOM intact / PERRLA / fundi: normal discs and vessels / icterus / exudate / hemorrhage

EARS EACs clear / TM translucent, mobile / landmarks abnormal / hearing diminished
NOSE lesions / mucosal inflammation / septum, turbinates abnormal / sinus tenderness
MOUTH mucous membranes dry / lesions / poor dentition / caries / gingival inflammation
PHARYNX mucosa inflammation / tonsillar hypertrophy / tonsillar exudate
NECK supple / ROM WNL / lesion / bruit / adenopathy / thyroid enlarged, tender / mass
CARDIAC regular rate, rhythm / S1, S2 / murmur / gallop / click / rub / PMI displacement
RESP clear to auscultation in all fields / wheezes (insp) (exp) / rales / crackles
ABDOMEN BSx4 / tender / organomegaly / mass / hernia
RECTAL abnormal tone / hemorrhoids (int/ext) / palpable mass
BACK abnormal curvature / tenderness / CVAT / Δ ROM
EXTREMITIES amputation / deformity / edema / varicosities / + pulses
MSK abnormal gait / asymmetry / crepitation / defect / tenderness / mass / effusion / Δ ROM / instability / atrophy / abnormal strength, tone in head, neck, spine, ribs, pelvis, UE, LE / pathologic reflexes

PSYCH A&O x3 / +recent/remote memory / insight / affect
BREAST nipple abnormality / mass / tenderness / axillary, clavicular adenopathy
GYN/GU lesions / d/c / uterus, adnexa tenderness / CMT // circumcised / penile lesions / urethra normal location, no d/c / testes normal / + cremasteric reflex
FEET + pulses / monofilament + / nails abnormal / dry, broken skin / callus

---

LABS CBC / CMP / lipids / TSH / microalbumin / A1C / UA, culture / PSA / iron studies / other:

DIAGNOSTICS XR / MRI / CT / US / cardiac / other
REFERRALS   **F/U** ___ wk ___ mo

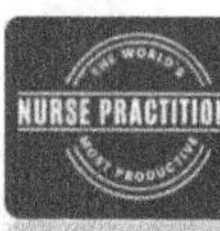

<table>
<tr><td colspan="2">
Patient ID#:   Date of visit:
Reason for visit: Age: Gender:
</td></tr>
</table>

BP: **HT:**
HR: **WT:**
T: **BMI:**
O2%:   **PAIN:**

NOTES . . . .

CONST	Δ appetite, energy, weight / fever / chills / sweats / fatigue
HEAD	trauma / mass / tenderness / rash / lesions
EYES	visionΔ / itch / d/c / tears / dry / cataracts / glaucoma / glasses, contacts
ENT	hearing Δ / pain / d/c / vertigo / ? infection // epistaxis / congestion // bleeding, swelling gums / pain / sore throat / voice Δ // neck pain / lumps / swelling / difficulty swallowing
CARDIAC	pain / pressure / dizzy / N / orthopnea / edema / palp / weak w exertion / hx murmurs / hx MI / HTN / HF / numb / tingle / cold extrem / slow wound healing
RESP	wheeze / SOB / cough / asthma / bronch / COPD
GI	abd pain / Δ in bowels / constipation / diarrhea / N V / hepatitis / gallstones / dysphagia / reflux / hemorrhoids / black, bloody stools
GU	burn / pain / nocturia / polyuria / hematuria / incontinence / infection / kid. stones
GENITAL	DC / sores / pain / masses / last pap ______ / sexually active Y N / dyspareunia / LMP ______ / contraception
MSK	redness / swelling / warmth / pain / +/- ROM / arthritis / musc cramps / fracture / sprains / joint replacement / stiffness: AM PM
SKIN	rash / pruritis / jaundice / bruising / hx skin ca / mole Δ / Δ in hair, nails / lesions / slow wound healing
BREASTS	lump / pain / dc / last mammo ______ / self exams YN
NEURO	HA / seizure / vertigo / memory Δ / gait Δ / speech / coord
PSYCH	depression / anxiety / Δ in sleep pattern / substance, ETOH abuse / suicidal ideation / homicidal ideation
ENDO	polydipsia, polyuria / heat, cold intolerance / Δ hair/nails/energy
HEM/LYMPH	anemia / bruising / hx transfusions / blood disorder / lymphadenopathy / axillary, groin tenderness
ALLX/IMMUN	season allx / food allx / med allx / immune disorder:

SOCIAL HX	# in household ______ / lives with SP/BF/GF/SO / children __ / tobacco Y/N #pk / sexual activity Y/N / etoh, other substances Y/N / occupation:
FAM HX	ca / HTN / MI / CAD / stroke / hyperlipidemia / DM2 / Alzheimer's / depression / osteoporosis / other:

GENERAL	well appearing / well nourished / a&o x 3 / normal mood / normal affect
NEURO	intact / abnormal **DTR:** 1 2 3 4 5 location:
SKIN + NAILS	turgor / rash / bruising / lesions // texture, distribution of hair // nails: abnormal color / nail deformity
HEAD	normocephalic / atraumatic / visible mass / palpable mass / depression / scarring
EYES	acuity intact / conjunctiva clear / EOM intact / PERRLA / fundi: normal discs and vessels / icterus / exudate / hemorrhage
EARS	EACs clear / TM translucent, mobile / landmarks abnormal / hearing diminished
NOSE	lesions / mucosal inflammation / septum, turbinates abnormal / sinus tenderness
MOUTH	mucous membranes dry / lesions / poor dentition / caries / gingival inflammation
PHARYNX	mucosa inflammation / tonsillar hypertrophy / tonsillar exudate
NECK	supple / ROM WNL / lesion / bruit / adenopathy / thyroid enlarged, tender / mass
CARDIAC	regular rate, rhythm / S1, S2 / murmur / gallop / click / rub / PMI displacement
RESP	clear to auscultation in all fields / wheezes (insp) (exp) / rales / crackles
ABDOMEN	BSx4 / tender / organomegaly / mass / hernia
RECTAL	abnormal tone / hemorrhoids (int/ext) / palpable mass
BACK	abnormal curvature / tenderness / CVAT / Δ ROM
EXTREMITIES	amputation / deformity / edema / varicosities / + pulses
MSK	abnormal gait / asymmetry / crepitation / defect / tenderness / mass / effusion / Δ ROM / instability / atrophy / abnormal strength, tone in head, neck, spine, ribs, pelvis, UE, LE / pathologic reflexes
PSYCH	A&O x3 / +recent/remote memory / insight / affect
BREAST	nipple abnormality / mass / tenderness / axillary, clavicular adenopathy
GYN/GU	lesions / d/c / uterus, adnexa tenderness / CMT // circumcised / penile lesions / urethra normal location, no d/c / testes normal / + cremasteric reflex
FEET	+ pulses / monofilament + / nails abnormal / dry, broken skin / callus

LABS	CBC / CMP / lipids / TSH / microalbumin / A1C / UA, culture / PSA / iron studies / other:

DIAGNOSTICS	XR / MRI / CT / US / cardiac / other
REFERRALS	**F/U** ___ wk ___ mo

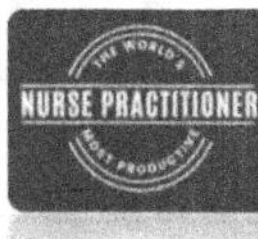

<table>
<tr><td>Patient ID#:</td><td>Date of visit:</td></tr>
<tr><td>Reason for visit:</td><td>Age: Gender:</td></tr>
</table>

BP:	HT:
HR:	WT:
T:	BMI:
O2%:	PAIN:

NOTES . . . .

CONST — Δ appetite, energy, weight / fever / chills / sweats / fatigue
HEAD — trauma / mass / tenderness / rash / lesions
EYES — visionΔ / itch / d/c / tears / dry / cataracts / glaucoma / glasses, contacts
ENT — hearing Δ / pain / d/c / vertigo / ? infection // epistaxis / congestion // bleeding, swelling gums / pain / sore throat / voice Δ // neck pain / lumps / swelling / difficulty swallowing

CARDIAC — pain / pressure / dizzy / N / orthopnea / edema / palp / weak w exertion / hx murmurs / hx MI / HTN / HF / numb / tingle / cold extrem / slow wound healing

RESP — wheeze / SOB / cough / asthma / bronch / COPD
GI — abd pain / Δ in bowels / constipation / diarrhea / N V / hepatitis / gallstones / dysphagia / reflux / hemorrhoids / black, bloody stools

GU — burn / pain / nocturia / polyuria / hematuria / incontinence / infection / kid. stones
GENITAL — DC / sores / pain / masses / last pap ______ / sexually active Y N / dyspareunia / LMP _______ / contraception

MSK — redness / swelling / warmth / pain / +/- ROM / arthritis / musc cramps / fracture / sprains / joint replacement / stiffness: AM PM

SKIN — rash / pruritis / jaundice / bruising / hx skin ca / mole Δ / Δ in hair, nails / lesions / slow wound healing

BREASTS — lump / pain / dc / last mammo _______ / self exams YN
NEURO — HA / seizure / vertigo / memory Δ / gait Δ / speech / coord
PSYCH — depression / anxiety / Δ in sleep pattern / substance, ETOH abuse / suicidal ideation / homicidal ideation

ENDO — polydipsia, polyuria / heat, cold intolerance / Δ hair/nails/energy
HEM/LYMPH — anemia / bruising / hx transfusions / blood disorder / lymphadenopathy / axillary, groin tenderness

ALLX/IMMUN — season allx / food allx / med allx / immune disorder:

SOCIAL HX — # in household ______ / lives with SP/BF/GF/SO / children __ / tobacco Y/N #pk / sexual activity Y/N / etoh, other substances Y/N / occupation:
FAM HX — ca / HTN / MI / CAD / stroke / hyperlipidemia / DM2 / Alzheimer's / depression / osteoporosis / other:

GENERAL — well appearing / well nourished / a&o x 3 / normal mood / normal affect
NEURO — intact / abnormal   **DTR:** 1 2 3 4 5 location:
SKIN + NAILS — turgor / rash / bruising / lesions // texture, distribution of hair // nails: abnormal color / nail deformity

HEAD — normocephalic / atraumatic / visible mass / palpable mass / depression / scarring
EYES — acuity intact / conjunctiva clear / EOM intact / PERRLA / fundi: normal discs and vessels / icterus / exudate / hemorrhage

EARS — EACs clear / TM translucent, mobile / landmarks abnormal / hearing diminished
NOSE — lesions / mucosal inflammation / septum, turbinates abnormal / sinus tenderness
MOUTH — mucous membranes dry / lesions / poor dentition / caries / gingival inflammation
PHARYNX — mucosa inflammation / tonsillar hypertrophy / tonsillar exudate
NECK — supple / ROM WNL / lesion / bruit / adenopathy / thyroid enlarged, tender / mass
CARDIAC — regular rate, rhythm / S1, S2 / murmur / gallop / click / rub / PMI displacement
RESP — clear to auscultation in all fields / wheezes (insp) (exp) / rales / crackles
ABDOMEN — BSx4 / tender / organomegaly / mass / hernia
RECTAL — abnormal tone / hemorrhoids (int/ext) / palpable mass
BACK — abnormal curvature / tenderness / CVAT / Δ ROM
EXTREMITIES — amputation / deformity / edema / varicosities / + pulses
MSK — abnormal gait / asymmetry / crepitation / defect / tenderness / mass / effusion / Δ ROM / instability / atrophy / abnormal strength, tone in head, neck, spine, ribs, pelvis, UE, LE / pathologic reflexes

PSYCH — A&O x3 / +recent/remote memory / insight / affect
BREAST — nipple abnormality / mass / tenderness / axillary, clavicular adenopathy
GYN/GU — lesions / d/c / uterus, adnexa tenderness / CMT // circumcised / penile lesions / urethra normal location, no d/c / testes normal / + cremasteric reflex
FEET — + pulses / monofilament + / nails abnormal / dry, broken skin / callus

---

LABS — CBC / CMP / lipids / TSH / microalbumin / A1C / UA, culture / PSA / iron studies / other:

DIAGNOSTICS — XR / MRI / CT / US / cardiac / other
REFERRALS —   **F/U** ___ wk ___ mo

BP:	HT:
HR:	WT:
T:	BMI:
O2%:	PAIN:

NOTES . . . .

| **Patient ID#:** | **Date of visit:** |
| **Reason for visit:** | **Age:** **Gender:** |

CONST   Δ appetite, energy, weight / fever / chills / sweats / fatigue

HEAD   trauma / mass / tenderness / rash / lesions

EYES   visionΔ / itch / d/c / tears / dry / cataracts / glaucoma / glasses, contacts

ENT   hearing Δ / pain / d/c / vertigo / ? infection // epistaxis / congestion // bleeding, swelling gums / pain / sore throat / voice Δ // neck pain / lumps / swelling / difficulty swallowing

CARDIAC   pain / pressure / dizzy / N / orthopnea / edema / palp / weak w exertion / hx murmurs / hx MI / HTN / HF / numb / tingle / cold extrem / slow wound healing

RESP   wheeze / SOB / cough / asthma / bronch / COPD

GI   abd pain / Δ in bowels / constipation / diarrhea / N V / hepatitis / gallstones / dysphagia / reflux / hemorrhoids / black, bloody stools

GU   burn / pain / nocturia / polyuria / hematuria / incontinence / infection / kid. stones

GENITAL   DC / sores / pain / masses / last pap _______ / sexually active Y N / dyspareunia / LMP _______ / contraception

MSK   redness / swelling / warmth / pain / +/- ROM / arthritis / musc cramps / fracture / sprains / joint replacement / stiffness: AM PM

SKIN   rash / pruritis / jaundice / bruising / hx skin ca / mole Δ / Δ in hair, nails / lesions / slow wound healing

BREASTS   lump / pain / dc / last mammo _______ / self exams YN

NEURO   HA / seizure / vertigo / memory Δ / gait Δ / speech / coord

PSYCH   depression / anxiety / Δ in sleep pattern / substance, ETOH abuse / suicidal ideation / homicidal ideation

ENDO   polydipsia, polyuria / heat, cold intolerance / Δ hair/nails/energy

HEM/LYMPH   anemia / bruising / hx transfusions / blood disorder / lymphadenopathy / axillary, groin tenderness

ALLX/IMMUN   season allx / food allx / med allx / immune disorder:

SOCIAL HX   # in household _______ / lives with SP/BF/GF/SO / children __ / tobacco Y/N #pk / sexual activity Y/N / etoh, other substances Y/N / occupation:

FAM HX   ca / HTN / MI / CAD / stroke / hyperlipidemia / DM2 / Alzheimer's / depression / osteoporosis / other:

GENERAL   well appearing / well nourished / a&o x 3 / normal mood / normal affect

NEURO   intact / abnormal   **DTR:** 1 2 3 4 5 location:

SKIN + NAILS   turgor / rash / bruising / lesions // texture, distribution of hair // nails: abnormal color / nail deformity

HEAD   normocephalic / atraumatic / visible mass / palpable mass / depression / scarring

EYES   acuity intact / conjunctiva clear / EOM intact / PERRLA / fundi: normal discs and vessels / icterus / exudate / hemorrhage

EARS   EACs clear / TM translucent, mobile / landmarks abnormal / hearing diminished

NOSE   lesions / mucosal inflammation / septum, turbinates abnormal / sinus tenderness

MOUTH   mucous membranes dry / lesions / poor dentition / caries / gingival inflammation

PHARYNX   mucosa inflammation / tonsillar hypertrophy / tonsillar exudate

NECK   supple / ROM WNL / lesion / bruit / adenopathy / thyroid enlarged, tender / mass

CARDIAC   regular rate, rhythm / S1, S2 / murmur / gallop / click / rub / PMI displacement

RESP   clear to auscultation in all fields / wheezes (insp) (exp) / rales / crackles

ABDOMEN   BSx4 / tender / organomegaly / mass / hernia

RECTAL   abnormal tone / hemorrhoids (int/ext) / palpable mass

BACK   abnormal curvature / tenderness / CVAT / Δ ROM

EXTREMITIES   amputation / deformity / edema / varicosities / + pulses

MSK   abnormal gait / asymmetry / crepitation / defect / tenderness / mass / effusion / Δ ROM / instability / atrophy / abnormal strength, tone in head, neck, spine, ribs, pelvis, UE, LE / pathologic reflexes

PSYCH   A&O x3 / +recent/remote memory / insight / affect

BREAST   nipple abnormality / mass / tenderness / axillary, clavicular adenopathy

GYN/GU   lesions / d/c / uterus, adnexa tenderness / CMT // circumcised / penile lesions / urethra normal location, no d/c / testes normal / + cremasteric reflex

FEET   + pulses / monofilament + / nails abnormal / dry, broken skin / callus

---

LABS   CBC / CMP / lipids / TSH / microalbumin / A1C / UA, culture / PSA / iron studies / other:

DIAGNOSTICS   XR / MRI / CT / US / cardiac / other

REFERRALS   **F/U** ___ wk ___ mo

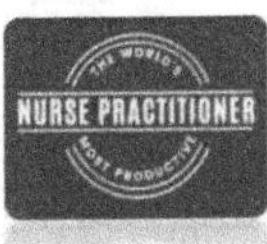

<table>
<tr><td colspan="2">
Patient ID#:
Reason for visit:
</td></tr>
<tr><td>
Date of visit:
Age: Gender:
</td></tr>
</table>

BP:	HT:
HR:	WT:
T:	BMI:
O2%:	PAIN:

NOTES . . . .

CONST Δ appetite, energy, weight / fever / chills / sweats / fatigue
HEAD trauma / mass / tenderness / rash / lesions
EYES visionΔ / itch / d/c / tears / dry / cataracts / glaucoma / glasses, contacts
ENT hearing Δ / pain / d/c / vertigo / ? infection // epistaxis / congestion // bleeding, swelling gums / pain / sore throat / voice Δ // neck pain / lumps / swelling / difficulty swallowing

CARDIAC pain / pressure / dizzy / N / orthopnea / edema / palp / weak w exertion / hx murmurs / hx MI / HTN / HF / numb / tingle / cold extrem / slow wound healing

RESP wheeze / SOB / cough / asthma / bronch / COPD
GI abd pain / Δ in bowels / constipation / diarrhea / N V / hepatitis / gallstones / dysphagia / reflux / hemorrhoids / black, bloody stools

GU burn / pain / nocturia / polyuria / hematuria / incontinence / infection / kid. stones
GENITAL DC / sores / pain / masses / last pap ______ / sexually active Y N / dyspareunia / LMP ______ / contraception

MSK redness / swelling / warmth / pain / +/- ROM / arthritis / musc cramps / fracture / sprains / joint replacement / stiffness: AM PM

SKIN rash / pruritis / jaundice / bruising / hx skin ca / mole Δ / Δ in hair, nails / lesions / slow wound healing

BREASTS lump / pain / dc / last mammo ______ / self exams YN
NEURO HA / seizure / vertigo / memory Δ / gait Δ / speech / coord
PSYCH depression / anxiety / Δ in sleep pattern / substance, ETOH abuse / suicidal ideation / homicidal ideation

ENDO polydipsia, polyuria / heat, cold intolerance / Δ hair/nails/energy
HEM/LYMPH anemia / bruising / hx transfusions / blood disorder / lymphadenopathy / axillary, groin tenderness
ALLX/IMMUN season allx / food allx / med allx / immune disorder:

SOCIAL HX # in household ______ / lives with SP/BF/GF/SO / children __ / tobacco Y/N #pk / sexual activity Y/N / etoh, other substances Y/N / occupation:
FAM HX ca / HTN / MI / CAD / stroke / hyperlipidemia / DM2 / Alzheimer's / depression / osteoporosis / other:

GENERAL well appearing / well nourished / a&o x 3 / normal mood / normal affect
NEURO intact / abnormal **DTR:** 1 2 3 4 5 location:
SKIN + NAILS turgor / rash / bruising / lesions // texture, distribution of hair // nails: abnormal color / nail deformity

HEAD normocephalic / atraumatic / visible mass / palpable mass / depression / scarring
EYES acuity intact / conjunctiva clear / EOM intact / PERRLA / fundi: normal discs and vessels / icterus / exudate / hemorrhage

EARS EACs clear / TM translucent, mobile / landmarks abnormal / hearing diminished
NOSE lesions / mucosal inflammation / septum, turbinates abnormal / sinus tenderness
MOUTH mucous membranes dry / lesions / poor dentition / caries / gingival inflammation
PHARYNX mucosa inflammation / tonsillar hypertrophy / tonsillar exudate
NECK supple / ROM WNL / lesion / bruit / adenopathy / thyroid enlarged, tender / mass
CARDIAC regular rate, rhythm / S1, S2 / murmur / gallop / click / rub / PMI displacement
RESP clear to auscultation in all fields / wheezes (insp) (exp) / rales / crackles
ABDOMEN BSx4 / tender / organomegaly / mass / hernia
RECTAL abnormal tone / hemorrhoids (int/ext) / palpable mass
BACK abnormal curvature / tenderness / CVAT / Δ ROM
EXTREMITIES amputation / deformity / edema / varicosities / + pulses
MSK abnormal gait / asymmetry / crepitation / defect / tenderness / mass / effusion / Δ ROM / instability / atrophy / abnormal strength, tone in head, neck, spine, ribs, pelvis, UE, LE / pathologic reflexes

PSYCH A&O x3 / +recent/remote memory / insight / affect
BREAST nipple abnormality / mass / tenderness / axillary, clavicular adenopathy
GYN/GU lesions / d/c / uterus, adnexa tenderness / CMT // circumcised / penile lesions / urethra normal location, no d/c / testes normal / + cremasteric reflex
FEET + pulses / monofilament + / nails abnormal / dry, broken skin / callus

---

LABS CBC / CMP / lipids / TSH / microalbumin / A1C / UA, culture / PSA / iron studies / other:

DIAGNOSTICS XR / MRI / CT / US / cardiac / other
REFERRALS

F/U ___ wk ___ mo

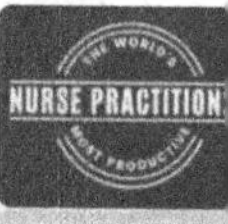

<table>
<tr><td colspan="2">Patient ID#:
Reason for visit:</td><td>Date of visit:
Age: Gender:</td></tr>
</table>

BP:	HT:
HR:	WT:
T:	BMI:
O2%:	PAIN:

NOTES . . . .

CONST	Δ appetite, energy, weight / fever / chills / sweats / fatigue
HEAD	trauma / mass / tenderness / rash / lesions
EYES	visionΔ / itch / d/c / tears / dry / cataracts / glaucoma / glasses, contacts
ENT	hearing Δ / pain / d/c / vertigo / ? infection // epistaxis / congestion // bleeding, swelling gums / pain / sore throat / voice Δ // neck pain / lumps / swelling / difficulty swallowing
CARDIAC	pain / pressure / dizzy / N / orthopnea / edema / palp / weak w exertion / hx murmurs / hx MI / HTN / HF / numb / tingle / cold extrem / slow wound healing
RESP	wheeze / SOB / cough / asthma / bronch / COPD
GI	abd pain / Δ in bowels / constipation / diarrhea / N V / hepatitis / gallstones / dysphagia / reflux / hemorrhoids / black, bloody stools
GU	burn / pain / nocturia / polyuria / hematuria / incontinence / infection / kid. stones
GENITAL	DC / sores / pain / masses / last pap ______ / sexually active Y N / dyspareunia / LMP ______ / contraception
MSK	redness / swelling / warmth / pain / +/- ROM / arthritis / musc cramps / fracture / sprains / joint replacement / stiffness: AM PM
SKIN	rash / pruritis / jaundice / bruising / hx skin ca / mole Δ / Δ in hair, nails / lesions / slow wound healing
BREASTS	lump / pain / dc / last mammo ______ / self exams YN
NEURO	HA / seizure / vertigo / memory Δ / gait Δ / speech / coord
PSYCH	depression / anxiety / Δ in sleep pattern / substance, ETOH abuse / suicidal ideation / homicidal ideation
ENDO	polydipsia, polyuria / heat, cold intolerance / Δ hair/nails/energy
HEM/LYMPH	anemia / bruising / hx transfusions / blood disorder / lymphadenopathy / axillary, groin tenderness
ALLX/IMMUN	season allx / food allx / med allx / immune disorder:

SOCIAL HX	# in household ______ / lives with SP/BF/GF/SO / children __ / tobacco Y/N #pk / sexual activity Y/N / etoh, other substances Y/N / occupation:
FAM HX	ca / HTN / MI / CAD / stroke / hyperlipidemia / DM2 / Alzheimer's / depression / osteoporosis / other:

GENERAL	well appearing / well nourished / a&o x 3 / normal mood / normal affect
NEURO	intact / abnormal **DTR:** 1 2 3 4 5 location:
SKIN + NAILS	turgor / rash / bruising / lesions // texture, distribution of hair // nails: abnormal color / nail deformity
HEAD	normocephalic / atraumatic / visible mass / palpable mass / depression / scarring
EYES	acuity intact / conjunctiva clear / EOM intact / PERRLA / fundi: normal discs and vessels / icterus / exudate / hemorrhage
EARS	EACs clear / TM translucent, mobile / landmarks abnormal / hearing diminished
NOSE	lesions / mucosal inflammation / septum, turbinates abnormal / sinus tenderness
MOUTH	mucous membranes dry / lesions / poor dentition / caries / gingival inflammation
PHARYNX	mucosa inflammation / tonsillar hypertrophy / tonsillar exudate
NECK	supple / ROM WNL / lesion / bruit / adenopathy / thyroid enlarged, tender / mass
CARDIAC	regular rate, rhythm / S1, S2 / murmur / gallop / click / rub / PMI displacement
RESP	clear to auscultation in all fields / wheezes (insp) (exp) / rales / crackles
ABDOMEN	BSx4 / tender / organomegaly / mass / hernia
RECTAL	abnormal tone / hemorrhoids (int/ext) / palpable mass
BACK	abnormal curvature / tenderness / CVAT / Δ ROM
EXTREMITIES	amputation / deformity / edema / varicosities / + pulses
MSK	abnormal gait / asymmetry / crepitation / defect / tenderness / mass / effusion / Δ ROM / instability / atrophy / abnormal strength, tone in head, neck, spine, ribs, pelvis, UE, LE / pathologic reflexes
PSYCH	A&O x3 / +recent/remote memory / insight / affect
BREAST	nipple abnormality / mass / tenderness / axillary, clavicular adenopathy
GYN/GU	lesions / d/c / uterus, adnexa tenderness / CMT // circumcised / penile lesions / urethra normal location, no d/c / testes normal / + cremasteric reflex
FEET	+ pulses / monofilament + / nails abnormal / dry, broken skin / callus

LABS	CBC / CMP / lipids / TSH / microalbumin / A1C / UA, culture / PSA / iron studies / other:

DIAGNOSTICS	XR / MRI / CT / US / cardiac / other
REFERRALS	**F/U** ___ wk ___ mo

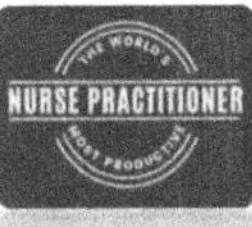

<table>
<tr><td>

Patient ID#:	Date of visit:
Reason for visit:	Age: Gender:

</td><td>

BP:	HT:
HR:	WT:
T:	BMI:
O2%:	PAIN:

NOTES . . . .

</td></tr>
</table>

CONST	Δ appetite, energy, weight / fever / chills / sweats / fatigue
HEAD	trauma / mass / tenderness / rash / lesions
EYES	visionΔ / itch / d/c / tears / dry / cataracts / glaucoma / glasses, contacts
ENT	hearing Δ / pain / d/c / vertigo / ? infection // epistaxis / congestion // bleeding, swelling gums / pain / sore throat / voice Δ // neck pain / lumps / swelling / difficulty swallowing
CARDIAC	pain / pressure / dizzy / N / orthopnea / edema / palp / weak w exertion / hx murmurs / hx MI / HTN / HF / numb / tingle / cold extrem / slow wound healing
RESP	wheeze / SOB / cough / asthma / bronch / COPD
GI	abd pain / Δ in bowels / constipation / diarrhea / N V / hepatitis / gallstones / dysphagia / reflux / hemorrhoids / black, bloody stools
GU	burn / pain / nocturia / polyuria / hematuria / incontinence / infection / kid. stones
GENITAL	DC / sores / pain / masses / last pap _____ / sexually active Y N / dyspareunia / LMP _____ / contraception
MSK	redness / swelling / warmth / pain / +/- ROM / arthritis / musc cramps / fracture / sprains / joint replacement / stiffness: AM PM
SKIN	rash / pruritis / jaundice / bruising / hx skin ca / mole Δ / Δ in hair, nails / lesions / slow wound healing
BREASTS	lump / pain / dc / last mammo _____ / self exams YN
NEURO	HA / seizure / vertigo / memory Δ / gait Δ / speech / coord
PSYCH	depression / anxiety / Δ in sleep pattern / substance, ETOH abuse / suicidal ideation / homicidal ideation
ENDO	polydipsia, polyuria / heat, cold intolerance / Δ hair/nails/energy
HEM/LYMPH	anemia / bruising / hx transfusions / blood disorder / lymphadenopathy / axillary, groin tenderness
ALLX/IMMUN	season allx / food allx / med allx / immune disorder:

SOCIAL HX	# in household _____ / lives with SP/BF/GF/SO / children __ / tobacco Y/N #pk / sexual activity Y/N / etoh, other substances Y/N / occupation:
FAM HX	ca / HTN / MI / CAD / stroke / hyperlipidemia / DM2 / Alzheimer's / depression / osteoporosis / other:

GENERAL	well appearing / well nourished / a&o x 3 / normal mood / normal affect
NEURO	intact / abnormal **DTR:** 1 2 3 4 5 location:
SKIN + NAILS	turgor / rash / bruising / lesions // texture, distribution of hair // nails: abnormal color / nail deformity
HEAD	normocephalic / atraumatic / visible mass / palpable mass / depression / scarring
EYES	acuity intact / conjunctiva clear / EOM intact / PERRLA / fundi: normal discs and vessels / icterus / exudate / hemorrhage
EARS	EACs clear / TM translucent, mobile / landmarks abnormal / hearing diminished
NOSE	lesions / mucosal inflammation / septum, turbinates abnormal / sinus tenderness
MOUTH	mucous membranes dry / lesions / poor dentition / caries / gingival inflammation
PHARYNX	mucosa inflammation / tonsillar hypertrophy / tonsillar exudate
NECK	supple / ROM WNL / lesion / bruit / adenopathy / thyroid enlarged, tender / mass
CARDIAC	regular rate, rhythm / S1, S2 / murmur / gallop / click / rub / PMI displacement
RESP	clear to auscultation in all fields / wheezes (insp) (exp) / rales / crackles
ABDOMEN	BSx4 / tender / organomegaly / mass / hernia
RECTAL	abnormal tone / hemorrhoids (int/ext) / palpable mass
BACK	abnormal curvature / tenderness / CVAT / Δ ROM
EXTREMITIES	amputation / deformity / edema / varicosities / + pulses
MSK	abnormal gait / asymmetry / crepitation / defect / tenderness / mass / effusion / Δ ROM / instability / atrophy / abnormal strength, tone in head, neck, spine, ribs, pelvis, UE, LE / pathologic reflexes
PSYCH	A&O x3 / +recent/remote memory / insight / affect
BREAST	nipple abnormality / mass / tenderness / axillary, clavicular adenopathy
GYN/GU	lesions / d/c / uterus, adnexa tenderness / CMT // circumcised / penile lesions / urethra normal location, no d/c / testes normal / + cremasteric reflex
FEET	+ pulses / monofilament + / nails abnormal / dry, broken skin / callus

LABS	CBC / CMP / lipids / TSH / microalbumin / A1C / UA, culture / PSA / iron studies / other:

DIAGNOSTICS	XR / MRI / CT / US / cardiac / other
REFERRALS	**F/U** ___ wk ___ mo

<table>
<tr><td>Patient ID#:</td><td>Date of visit:</td></tr>
<tr><td>Reason for visit:</td><td>Age: Gender:</td></tr>
</table>

BP: HT:
HR: WT:
T: BMI:
O2%:   PAIN:

NOTES . . . .

CONST Δ appetite, energy, weight / fever / chills / sweats / fatigue
HEAD trauma / mass / tenderness / rash / lesions
EYES visionΔ / itch / d/c / tears / dry / cataracts / glaucoma / glasses, contacts
ENT hearing Δ / pain / d/c / vertigo / ? infection // epistaxis / congestion // bleeding, swelling gums / pain / sore throat / voice Δ // neck pain / lumps / swelling / difficulty swallowing

CARDIAC pain / pressure / dizzy / N / orthopnea / edema / palp / weak w exertion / hx murmurs / hx MI / HTN / HF / numb / tingle / cold extrem / slow wound healing

RESP wheeze / SOB / cough / asthma / bronch / COPD
GI abd pain / Δ in bowels / constipation / diarrhea / N V / hepatitis / gallstones / dysphagia / reflux / hemorrhoids / black, bloody stools

GU burn / pain / nocturia / polyuria / hematuria / incontinence / infection / kid. stones
GENITAL DC / sores / pain / masses / last pap ______ / sexually active Y N / dyspareunia / LMP ______ / contraception

MSK redness / swelling / warmth / pain / +/- ROM / arthritis / musc cramps / fracture / sprains / joint replacement / stiffness: AM PM
SKIN rash / pruritis / jaundice / bruising / hx skin ca / mole Δ / Δ in hair, nails / lesions / slow wound healing

BREASTS lump / pain / dc / last mammo ______ / self exams YN
NEURO HA / seizure / vertigo / memory Δ / gait Δ / speech / coord
PSYCH depression / anxiety / Δ in sleep pattern / substance, ETOH abuse / suicidal ideation / homicidal ideation

ENDO polydipsia, polyuria / heat, cold intolerance / Δ hair/nails/energy
HEM/LYMPH anemia / bruising / hx transfusions / blood disorder / lymphadenopathy / axillary, groin tenderness

ALLX/IMMUN season allx / food allx / med allx / immune disorder:

SOCIAL HX # in household ______ / lives with SP/BF/GF/SO / children __ / tobacco Y/N #pk / sexual activity Y/N / etoh, other substances Y/N / occupation:
FAM HX ca / HTN / MI / CAD / stroke / hyperlipidemia / DM2 / Alzheimer's / depression / osteoporosis / other:

GENERAL well appearing / well nourished / a&o x 3 / normal mood / normal affect
NEURO intact / abnormal   **DTR:** 1 2 3 4 5 location:
SKIN + NAILS turgor / rash / bruising / lesions // texture, distribution of hair // nails: abnormal color / nail deformity

HEAD normocephalic / atraumatic / visible mass / palpable mass / depression / scarring
EYES acuity intact / conjunctiva clear / EOM intact / PERRLA / fundi: normal discs and vessels / icterus / exudate / hemorrhage

EARS EACs clear / TM translucent, mobile / landmarks abnormal / hearing diminished
NOSE lesions / mucosal inflammation / septum, turbinates abnormal / sinus tenderness
MOUTH mucous membranes dry / lesions / poor dentition / caries / gingival inflammation
PHARYNX mucosa inflammation / tonsillar hypertrophy / tonsillar exudate
NECK supple / ROM WNL / lesion / bruit / adenopathy / thyroid enlarged, tender / mass
CARDIAC regular rate, rhythm / S1, S2 / murmur / gallop / click / rub / PMI displacement
RESP clear to auscultation in all fields / wheezes (insp) (exp) / rales / crackles
ABDOMEN BSx4 / tender / organomegaly / mass / hernia
RECTAL abnormal tone / hemorrhoids (int/ext) / palpable mass
BACK abnormal curvature / tenderness / CVAT / Δ ROM
EXTREMITIES amputation / deformity / edema / varicosities / + pulses
MSK abnormal gait / asymmetry / crepitation / defect / tenderness / mass / effusion / Δ ROM / instability / atrophy / abnormal strength, tone in head, neck, spine, ribs, pelvis, UE, LE / pathologic reflexes

PSYCH A&O x3 / +recent/remote memory / insight / affect
BREAST nipple abnormality / mass / tenderness / axillary, clavicular adenopathy
GYN/GU lesions / d/c / uterus, adnexa tenderness / CMT // circumcised / penile lesions / urethra normal location, no d/c / testes normal / + cremasteric reflex
FEET + pulses / monofilament + / nails abnormal / dry, broken skin / callus

LABS CBC / CMP / lipids / TSH / microalbumin / A1C / UA, culture / PSA / iron studies / other:

DIAGNOSTICS XR / MRI / CT / US / cardiac / other
REFERRALS   **F/U** ___ wk ___ mo

<table>
<tr><td>

Patient ID#:	Date of visit:
Reason for visit:	Age: Gender:

</td><td>

BP:	HT:
HR:	WT:
T:	BMI:
O2%:	PAIN:

NOTES . . . .

</td></tr>
</table>

CONST — Δ appetite, energy, weight / fever / chills / sweats / fatigue
HEAD — trauma / mass / tenderness / rash / lesions
EYES — visionΔ / itch / d/c / tears / dry / cataracts / glaucoma / glasses, contacts
ENT — hearing Δ / pain / d/c / vertigo / ? infection *II* epistaxis / congestion *II* bleeding, swelling gums / pain / sore throat / voice Δ *II* neck pain / lumps / swelling / difficulty swallowing

CARDIAC — pain / pressure / dizzy / N / orthopnea / edema / palp / weak w exertion / hx murmurs / hx MI / HTN / HF / numb / tingle / cold extrem / slow wound healing

RESP — wheeze / SOB / cough / asthma / bronch / COPD
GI — abd pain / Δ in bowels / constipation / diarrhea / N V / hepatitis / gallstones / dysphagia / reflux / hemorrhoids / black, bloody stools

GU — burn / pain / nocturia / polyuria / hematuria / incontinence / infection / kid. stones
GENITAL — DC / sores / pain / masses / last pap _____ / sexually active Y N / dyspareunia / LMP _______ / contraception

MSK — redness / swelling / warmth / pain / +/- ROM / arthritis / musc cramps / fracture / sprains / joint replacement / stiffness: AM PM

SKIN — rash / pruritis / jaundice / bruising / hx skin ca / mole Δ / Δ in hair, nails / lesions / slow wound healing

BREASTS — lump / pain / dc / last mammo _____ / self exams YN
NEURO — HA / seizure / vertigo / memory Δ / gait Δ / speech / coord
PSYCH — depression / anxiety / Δ in sleep pattern / substance, ETOH abuse / suicidal ideation / homicidal ideation

ENDO — polydipsia, polyuria / heat, cold intolerance / Δ hair/nails/energy
HEM/LYMPH — anemia / bruising / hx transfusions / blood disorder / lymphadenopathy / axillary, groin tenderness

ALLX/IMMUN — season allx / food allx / med allx / immune disorder:

SOCIAL HX — # in household _______ / lives with SP/BF/GF/SO / children __ / tobacco Y/N #pk / sexual activity Y/N / etoh, other substances Y/N / occupation:

FAM HX — ca / HTN / MI / CAD / stroke / hyperlipidemia / DM2 / Alzheimer's / depression / osteoporosis / other:

GENERAL — well appearing / well nourished / a&o x 3 / normal mood / normal affect
NEURO — intact / abnormal   **DTR:** 1 2 3 4 5 location:
SKIN + NAILS — turgor / rash / bruising / lesions *II* texture, distribution of hair *II* nails: abnormal color / nail deformity

HEAD — normocephalic / atraumatic / visible mass / palpable mass / depression / scarring
EYES — acuity intact / conjunctiva clear / EOM intact / PERRLA / fundi: normal discs and vessels / icterus / exudate / hemorrhage

EARS — EACs clear / TM translucent, mobile / landmarks abnormal / hearing diminished
NOSE — lesions / mucosal inflammation / septum, turbinates abnormal / sinus tenderness
MOUTH — mucous membranes dry / lesions / poor dentition / caries / gingival inflammation
PHARYNX — mucosa inflammation / tonsillar hypertrophy / tonsillar exudate
NECK — supple / ROM WNL / lesion / bruit / adenopathy / thyroid enlarged, tender / mass
CARDIAC — regular rate, rhythm / S1, S2 / murmur / gallop / click / rub / PMI displacement
RESP — clear to auscultation in all fields / wheezes (insp) (exp) / rales / crackles
ABDOMEN — BSx4 / tender / organomegaly / mass / hernia
RECTAL — abnormal tone / hemorrhoids (int/ext) / palpable mass
BACK — abnormal curvature / tenderness / CVAT / Δ ROM
EXTREMITIES — amputation / deformity / edema / varicosities / + pulses
MSK — abnormal gait / asymmetry / crepitation / defect / tenderness / mass / effusion / Δ ROM / instability / atrophy / abnormal strength, tone in head, neck, spine, ribs, pelvis, UE, LE / pathologic reflexes

PSYCH — A&O x3 / +recent/remote memory / insight / affect
BREAST — nipple abnormality / mass / tenderness / axillary, clavicular adenopathy
GYN/GU — lesions / d/c / uterus, adnexa tenderness / CMT *II* circumcised / penile lesions / urethra normal location, no d/c / testes normal / + cremasteric reflex

FEET — + pulses / monofilament + / nails abnormal / dry, broken skin / callus

---

LABS — CBC / CMP / lipids / TSH / microalbumin / A1C / UA, culture / PSA / iron studies / other:

DIAGNOSTICS — XR / MRI / CT / US / cardiac / other
REFERRALS —   **F/U** ___ wk ___ mo

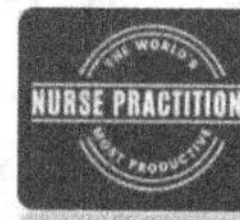

<table>
<tr><td>BP:</td><td>HT:</td></tr>
<tr><td>HR:</td><td>WT:</td></tr>
<tr><td>T:</td><td>BMI:</td></tr>
<tr><td>O2%:</td><td>PAIN:</td></tr>
</table>

CONST	Δ appetite, energy, weight / fever / chills / sweats / fatigue
HEAD	trauma / mass / tenderness / rash / lesions
EYES	visionΔ / itch / d/c / tears / dry / cataracts / glaucoma / glasses, contacts
ENT	hearing Δ / pain / d/c / vertigo / ? infection // epistaxis / congestion // bleeding, swelling gums / pain / sore throat / voice Δ // neck pain / lumps / swelling / difficulty swallowing
CARDIAC	pain / pressure / dizzy / N / orthopnea / edema / palp / weak w exertion / hx murmurs / hx MI / HTN / HF / numb / tingle / cold extrem / slow wound healing
RESP	wheeze / SOB / cough / asthma / bronch / COPD
GI	abd pain / Δ in bowels / constipation / diarrhea / N V / hepatitis / gallstones / dysphagia / reflux / hemorrhoids / black, bloody stools
GU	burn / pain / nocturia / polyuria / hematuria / incontinence / infection / kid. stones
GENITAL	DC / sores / pain / masses / last pap _____ / sexually active Y N / dyspareunia / LMP _______ / contraception
MSK	redness / swelling / warmth / pain / +/- ROM / arthritis / musc cramps / fracture / sprains / joint replacement / stiffness: AM PM
SKIN	rash / pruritis / jaundice / bruising / hx skin ca / mole Δ / Δ in hair, nails / lesions / slow wound healing
BREASTS	lump / pain / dc / last mammo ______ / self exams YN
NEURO	HA / seizure / vertigo / memory Δ / gait Δ / speech / coord
PSYCH	depression / anxiety / Δ in sleep pattern / substance, ETOH abuse / suicidal ideation / homicidal ideation
ENDO	polydipsia, polyuria / heat, cold intolerance / Δ hair/nails/energy
HEM/LYMPH	anemia / bruising / hx transfusions / blood disorder / lymphadenopathy / axillary, groin tenderness
ALLX/IMMUN	season allx / food allx / med allx / immune disorder:

SOCIAL HX	# in household _____ / lives with SP/BF/GF/SO / children __ / tobacco Y/N #pk / sexual activity Y/N / etoh, other substances Y/N / occupation:
FAM HX	ca / HTN / MI / CAD / stroke / hyperlipidemia / DM2 / Alzheimer's / depression / osteoporosis / other:

GENERAL	well appearing / well nourished / a&o x 3 / normal mood / normal affect
NEURO	intact / abnormal **DTR:** 1 2 3 4 5 location:
SKIN + NAILS	turgor / rash / bruising / lesions // texture, distribution of hair // nails: abnormal color / nail deformity
HEAD	normocephalic / atraumatic / visible mass / palpable mass / depression / scarring
EYES	acuity intact / conjunctiva clear / EOM intact / PERRLA / fundi: normal discs and vessels / icterus / exudate / hemorrhage
EARS	EACs clear / TM translucent, mobile / landmarks abnormal / hearing diminished
NOSE	lesions / mucosal inflammation / septum, turbinates abnormal / sinus tenderness
MOUTH	mucous membranes dry / lesions / poor dentition / caries / gingival inflammation
PHARYNX	mucosa inflammation / tonsillar hypertrophy / tonsillar exudate
NECK	supple / ROM WNL / lesion / bruit / adenopathy / thyroid enlarged, tender / mass
CARDIAC	regular rate, rhythm / S1, S2 / murmur / gallop / click / rub / PMI displacement
RESP	clear to auscultation in all fields / wheezes (insp) (exp) / rales / crackles
ABDOMEN	BSx4 / tender / organomegaly / mass / hernia
RECTAL	abnormal tone / hemorrhoids (int/ext) / palpable mass
BACK	abnormal curvature / tenderness / CVAT / Δ ROM
EXTREMITIES	amputation / deformity / edema / varicosities / + pulses
MSK	abnormal gait / asymmetry / crepitation / defect / tenderness / mass / effusion / Δ ROM / instability / atrophy / abnormal strength, tone in head, neck, spine, ribs, pelvis, UE, LE / pathologic reflexes
PSYCH	A&O x3 / +recent/remote memory / insight / affect
BREAST	nipple abnormality / mass / tenderness / axillary, clavicular adenopathy
GYN/GU	lesions / d/c / uterus, adnexa tenderness / CMT // circumcised / penile lesions / urethra normal location, no d/c / testes normal / + cremasteric reflex
FEET	+ pulses / monofilament + / nails abnormal / dry, broken skin / callus

LABS	CBC / CMP / lipids / TSH / microalbumin / A1C / UA, culture / PSA / iron studies / other:

DIAGNOSTICS	XR / MRI / CT / US / cardiac / other
REFERRALS	**F/U** ___ wk ___ mo

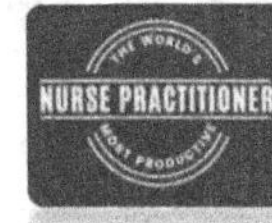

<table>
<tr><td>

Patient ID#:

Reason for visit:
</td><td>

Date of visit:

Age: **Gender:**
</td></tr>
</table>

BP:	HT:
HR:	WT:
T:	BMI:
O2%:	PAIN:

NOTES . . . .

CONST	Δ appetite, energy, weight / fever / chills / sweats / fatigue
HEAD	trauma / mass / tenderness / rash / lesions
EYES	visionΔ / itch / d/c / tears / dry / cataracts / glaucoma / glasses, contacts
ENT	hearing Δ / pain / d/c / vertigo / ? infection // epistaxis / congestion // bleeding, swelling gums / pain / sore throat / voice Δ // neck pain / lumps / swelling / difficulty swallowing
CARDIAC	pain / pressure / dizzy / N / orthopnea / edema / palp / weak w exertion / hx murmurs / hx MI / HTN / HF / numb / tingle / cold extrem / slow wound healing
RESP	wheeze / SOB / cough / asthma / bronch / COPD
GI	abd pain / Δ in bowels / constipation / diarrhea / N V / hepatitis / gallstones / dysphagia / reflux / hemorrhoids / black, bloody stools
GU	burn / pain / nocturia / polyuria / hematuria / incontinence / infection / kid. stones
GENITAL	DC / sores / pain / masses / last pap _____ / sexually active Y N / dyspareunia / LMP _____ / contraception
MSK	redness / swelling / warmth / pain / +/- ROM / arthritis / musc cramps / fracture / sprains / joint replacement / stiffness: AM PM
SKIN	rash / pruritis / jaundice / bruising / hx skin ca / mole Δ / Δ in hair, nails / lesions / slow wound healing
BREASTS	lump / pain / dc / last mammo _____ / self exams YN
NEURO	HA / seizure / vertigo / memory Δ / gait Δ / speech / coord
PSYCH	depression / anxiety / Δ in sleep pattern / substance, ETOH abuse / suicidal ideation / homicidal ideation
ENDO	polydipsia, polyuria / heat, cold intolerance / Δ hair/nails/energy
HEM/LYMPH	anemia / bruising / hx transfusions / blood disorder / lymphadenopathy / axillary, groin tenderness
ALLX/IMMUN	season allx / food allx / med allx / immune disorder:

SOCIAL HX	# in household _____ / lives with SP/BF/GF/SO / children __ / tobacco Y/N #pk / sexual activity Y/N / etoh, other substances Y/N / occupation:
FAM HX	ca / HTN / MI / CAD / stroke / hyperlipidemia / DM2 / Alzheimer's / depression / osteoporosis / other:

GENERAL	well appearing / well nourished / a&o x 3 / normal mood / normal affect
NEURO	intact / abnormal **DTR:** 1 2 3 4 5 location:
SKIN + NAILS	turgor / rash / bruising / lesions // texture, distribution of hair // nails: abnormal color / nail deformity
HEAD	normocephalic / atraumatic / visible mass / palpable mass / depression / scarring
EYES	acuity intact / conjunctiva clear / EOM intact / PERRLA / fundi: normal discs and vessels / icterus / exudate / hemorrhage
EARS	EACs clear / TM translucent, mobile / landmarks abnormal / hearing diminished
NOSE	lesions / mucosal inflammation / septum, turbinates abnormal / sinus tenderness
MOUTH	mucous membranes dry / lesions / poor dentition / caries / gingival inflammation
PHARYNX	mucosa inflammation / tonsillar hypertrophy / tonsillar exudate
NECK	supple / ROM WNL / lesion / bruit / adenopathy / thyroid enlarged, tender / mass
CARDIAC	regular rate, rhythm / S1, S2 / murmur / gallop / click / rub / PMI displacement
RESP	clear to auscultation in all fields / wheezes (insp) (exp) / rales / crackles
ABDOMEN	BSx4 / tender / organomegaly / mass / hernia
RECTAL	abnormal tone / hemorrhoids (int/ext) / palpable mass
BACK	abnormal curvature / tenderness / CVAT / Δ ROM
EXTREMITIES	amputation / deformity / edema / varicosities / + pulses
MSK	abnormal gait / asymmetry / crepitation / defect / tenderness / mass / effusion / Δ ROM / instability / atrophy / abnormal strength, tone in head, neck, spine, ribs, pelvis, UE, LE / pathologic reflexes
PSYCH	A&O x3 / +recent/remote memory / insight / affect
BREAST	nipple abnormality / mass / tenderness / axillary, clavicular adenopathy
GYN/GU	lesions / d/c / uterus, adnexa tenderness / CMT // circumcised / penile lesions / urethra normal location, no d/c / testes normal / + cremasteric reflex
FEET	+ pulses / monofilament + / nails abnormal / dry, broken skin / callus

LABS	CBC / CMP / lipids / TSH / microalbumin / A1C / UA, culture / PSA / iron studies / other:

DIAGNOSTICS	XR / MRI / CT / US / cardiac / other
REFERRALS	**F/U** ___ wk ___ mo

<table>
<tr><td colspan="2">

Patient ID#:   **Date of visit:**
Reason for visit: **Age:**   **Gender:**

</td><td>

BP: **HT:**
HR: **WT:**
T: **BMI:**
O2%:   **PAIN:**

</td></tr>
</table>

NOTES . . . .

CONST	Δ appetite, energy, weight / fever / chills / sweats / fatigue
HEAD	trauma / mass / tenderness / rash / lesions
EYES	visionΔ / itch / d/c / tears / dry / cataracts / glaucoma / glasses, contacts
ENT	hearing Δ / pain / d/c / vertigo / ? infection // epistaxis / congestion // bleeding, swelling gums / pain / sore throat / voice Δ // neck pain / lumps / swelling / difficulty swallowing
CARDIAC	pain / pressure / dizzy / N / orthopnea / edema / palp / weak w exertion / hx murmurs / hx MI / HTN / HF / numb / tingle / cold extrem / slow wound healing
RESP	wheeze / SOB / cough / asthma / bronch / COPD
GI	abd pain / Δ in bowels / constipation / diarrhea / N V / hepatitis / gallstones / dysphagia / reflux / hemorrhoids / black, bloody stools
GU	burn / pain / nocturia / polyuria / hematuria / incontinence / infection / kid. stones
GENITAL	DC / sores / pain / masses / last pap _____ / sexually active Y N / dyspareunia / LMP _____ / contraception
MSK	redness / swelling / warmth / pain / +/- ROM / arthritis / musc cramps / fracture / sprains / joint replacement / stiffness: AM PM
SKIN	rash / pruritis / jaundice / bruising / hx skin ca / mole Δ / Δ in hair, nails / lesions / slow wound healing
BREASTS	lump / pain / dc / last mammo _____ / self exams YN
NEURO	HA / seizure / vertigo / memory Δ / gait Δ / speech / coord
PSYCH	depression / anxiety / Δ in sleep pattern / substance, ETOH abuse / suicidal ideation / homicidal ideation
ENDO	polydipsia, polyuria / heat, cold intolerance / Δ hair/nails/energy
HEM/LYMPH	anemia / bruising / hx transfusions / blood disorder / lymphadenopathy / axillary, groin tenderness
ALLX/IMMUN	season allx / food allx / med allx / immune disorder:
SOCIAL HX	# in household _____ / lives with SP/BF/GF/SO / children __ / tobacco Y/N #pk / sexual activity Y/N / etoh, other substances Y/N / occupation:
FAM HX	ca / HTN / MI / CAD / stroke / hyperlipidemia / DM2 / Alzheimer's / depression / osteoporosis / other:
GENERAL	well appearing / well nourished / a&o x 3 / normal mood / normal affect
NEURO	intact / abnormal **DTR:** 1 2 3 4 5 location:
SKIN + NAILS	turgor / rash / bruising / lesions // texture, distribution of hair // nails: abnormal color / nail deformity
HEAD	normocephalic / atraumatic / visible mass / palpable mass / depression / scarring
EYES	acuity intact / conjunctiva clear / EOM intact / PERRLA / fundi: normal discs and vessels / icterus / exudate / hemorrhage
EARS	EACs clear / TM translucent, mobile / landmarks abnormal / hearing diminished
NOSE	lesions / mucosal inflammation / septum, turbinates abnormal / sinus tenderness
MOUTH	mucous membranes dry / lesions / poor dentition / caries / gingival inflammation
PHARYNX	mucosa inflammation / tonsillar hypertrophy / tonsillar exudate
NECK	supple / ROM WNL / lesion / bruit / adenopathy / thyroid enlarged, tender / mass
CARDIAC	regular rate, rhythm / S1, S2 / murmur / gallop / click / rub / PMI displacement
RESP	clear to auscultation in all fields / wheezes (insp) (exp) / rales / crackles
ABDOMEN	BSx4 / tender / organomegaly / mass / hernia
RECTAL	abnormal tone / hemorrhoids (int/ext) / palpable mass
BACK	abnormal curvature / tenderness / CVAT / Δ ROM
EXTREMITIES	amputation / deformity / edema / varicosities / + pulses
MSK	abnormal gait / asymmetry / crepitation / defect / tenderness / mass / effusion / Δ ROM / instability / atrophy / abnormal strength, tone in head, neck, spine, ribs, pelvis, UE, LE / pathologic reflexes
PSYCH	A&O x3 / +recent/remote memory / insight / affect
BREAST	nipple abnormality / mass / tenderness / axillary, clavicular adenopathy
GYN/GU	lesions / d/c / uterus, adnexa tenderness / CMT // circumcised / penile lesions / urethra normal location, no d/c / testes normal / + cremasteric reflex
FEET	+ pulses / monofilament + / nails abnormal / dry, broken skin / callus
LABS	CBC / CMP / lipids / TSH / microalbumin / A1C / UA, culture / PSA / iron studies / other:
DIAGNOSTICS	XR / MRI / CT / US / cardiac / other
REFERRALS	**F/U** ___ wk ___ mo

<table>
<tr><td colspan="2">

Patient ID#: 　　　　　　　　　　Date of visit:

Reason for visit: 　　　　　　　　Age:　　Gender:

</td><td>

BP: 　　　　　　HT:

HR: 　　　　　　WT:

T: 　　　　　　BMI:

O2%: 　　　　　PAIN:

</td></tr>
</table>

NOTES . . . .

CONST	Δ appetite, energy, weight / fever / chills / sweats / fatigue
HEAD	trauma / mass / tenderness / rash / lesions
EYES	visionΔ / itch / d/c / tears / dry / cataracts / glaucoma / glasses, contacts
ENT	hearing Δ / pain / d/c / vertigo / ? infection // epistaxis / congestion // bleeding, swelling gums / pain / sore throat / voice Δ // neck pain / lumps / swelling / difficulty swallowing
CARDIAC	pain / pressure / dizzy / N / orthopnea / edema / palp / weak w exertion / hx murmurs / hx MI / HTN / HF / numb / tingle / cold extrem / slow wound healing
RESP	wheeze / SOB / cough / asthma / bronch / COPD
GI	abd pain / Δ in bowels / constipation / diarrhea / N V / hepatitis / gallstones / dysphagia / reflux / hemorrhoids / black, bloody stools
GU	burn / pain / nocturia / polyuria / hematuria / incontinence / infection / kid. stones
GENITAL	DC / sores / pain / masses / last pap _____ / sexually active Y N / dyspareunia / LMP _____ / contraception
MSK	redness / swelling / warmth / pain / +/- ROM / arthritis / musc cramps / fracture / sprains / joint replacement / stiffness: AM PM
SKIN	rash / pruritis / jaundice / bruising / hx skin ca / mole Δ / Δ in hair, nails / lesions / slow wound healing
BREASTS	lump / pain / dc / last mammo _____ / self exams YN
NEURO	HA / seizure / vertigo / memory Δ / gait Δ / speech / coord
PSYCH	depression / anxiety / Δ in sleep pattern / substance, ETOH abuse / suicidal ideation / homicidal ideation
ENDO	polydipsia, polyuria / heat, cold intolerance / Δ hair/nails/energy
HEM/LYMPH	anemia / bruising / hx transfusions / blood disorder / lymphadenopathy / axillary, groin tenderness
ALLX/IMMUN	season allx / food allx / med allx / immune disorder:

SOCIAL HX	# in household _____ / lives with SP/BF/GF/SO / children __ / tobacco Y/N #pk / sexual activity Y/N / etoh, other substances Y/N / occupation:
FAM HX	ca / HTN / MI / CAD / stroke / hyperlipidemia / DM2 / Alzheimer's / depression / osteoporosis / other:

GENERAL	well appearing / well nourished / a&o x 3 / normal mood / normal affect
NEURO	intact / abnormal 　　　　　　**DTR:** 1 2 3 4 5 location:
SKIN + NAILS	turgor / rash / bruising / lesions // texture, distribution of hair // nails: abnormal color / nail deformity
HEAD	normocephalic / atraumatic / visible mass / palpable mass / depression / scarring
EYES	acuity intact / conjunctiva clear / EOM intact / PERRLA / fundi: normal discs and vessels / icterus / exudate / hemorrhage
EARS	EACs clear / TM translucent, mobile / landmarks abnormal / hearing diminished
NOSE	lesions / mucosal inflammation / septum, turbinates abnormal / sinus tenderness
MOUTH	mucous membranes dry / lesions / poor dentition / caries / gingival inflammation
PHARYNX	mucosa inflammation / tonsillar hypertrophy / tonsillar exudate
NECK	supple / ROM WNL / lesion / bruit / adenopathy / thyroid enlarged, tender / mass
CARDIAC	regular rate, rhythm / S1, S2 / murmur / gallop / click / rub / PMI displacement
RESP	clear to auscultation in all fields / wheezes (insp) (exp) / rales / crackles
ABDOMEN	BSx4 / tender / organomegaly / mass / hernia
RECTAL	abnormal tone / hemorrhoids (int/ext) / palpable mass
BACK	abnormal curvature / tenderness / CVAT / Δ ROM
EXTREMITIES	amputation / deformity / edema / varicosities / + pulses
MSK	abnormal gait / asymmetry / crepitation / defect / tenderness / mass / effusion / Δ ROM / instability / atrophy / abnormal strength, tone in head, neck, spine, ribs, pelvis, UE, LE / pathologic reflexes
PSYCH	A&O x3 / +recent/remote memory / insight / affect
BREAST	nipple abnormality / mass / tenderness / axillary, clavicular adenopathy
GYN/GU	lesions / d/c / uterus, adnexa tenderness / CMT // circumcised / penile lesions / urethra normal location, no d/c / testes normal / + cremasteric reflex
FEET	+ pulses / monofilament + / nails abnormal / dry, broken skin / callus

LABS	CBC / CMP / lipids / TSH / microalbumin / A1C / UA, culture / PSA / iron studies / other:

DIAGNOSTICS	XR / MRI / CT / US / cardiac / other
REFERRALS	**F/U** ___ wk ___ mo

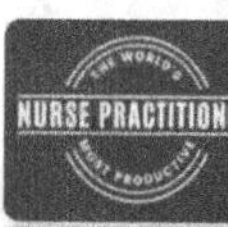

<table>
<tr><td colspan="2">

Patient ID#:   **Date of visit:**
Reason for visit: **Age:**   **Gender:**

</td></tr>
</table>

BP: **HT:**
HR: **WT:**
T: **BMI:**
O2%:   **PAIN:**

NOTES . . . .

CONST	Δ appetite, energy, weight / fever / chills / sweats / fatigue
HEAD	trauma / mass / tenderness / rash / lesions
EYES	visionΔ / itch / d/c / tears / dry / cataracts / glaucoma / glasses, contacts
ENT	hearing Δ / pain / d/c / vertigo / ? infection // epistaxis / congestion // bleeding, swelling gums / pain / sore throat / voice Δ // neck pain / lumps / swelling / difficulty swallowing
CARDIAC	pain / pressure / dizzy / N / orthopnea / edema / palp / weak w exertion / hx murmurs / hx MI / HTN / HF / numb / tingle / cold extrem / slow wound healing
RESP	wheeze / SOB / cough / asthma / bronch / COPD
GI	abd pain / Δ in bowels / constipation / diarrhea / N V / hepatitis / gallstones / dysphagia / reflux / hemorrhoids / black, bloody stools
GU	burn / pain / nocturia / polyuria / hematuria / incontinence / infection / kid. stones
GENITAL	DC / sores / pain / masses / last pap ______ / sexually active Y N / dyspareunia / LMP ______ / contraception
MSK	redness / swelling / warmth / pain / +/- ROM / arthritis / musc cramps / fracture / sprains / joint replacement / stiffness: AM PM
SKIN	rash / pruritis / jaundice / bruising / hx skin ca / mole Δ / Δ in hair, nails / lesions / slow wound healing
BREASTS	lump / pain / dc / last mammo ______ / self exams YN
NEURO	HA / seizure / vertigo / memory Δ / gait Δ / speech / coord
PSYCH	depression / anxiety / Δ in sleep pattern / substance, ETOH abuse / suicidal ideation / homicidal ideation
ENDO	polydipsia, polyuria / heat, cold intolerance / Δ hair/nails/energy
HEM/LYMPH	anemia / bruising / hx transfusions / blood disorder / lymphadenopathy / axillary, groin tenderness
ALLX/IMMUN	season allx / food allx / med allx / immune disorder:

SOCIAL HX	# in household ______ / lives with SP/BF/GF/SO / children __ / tobacco Y/N #pk / sexual activity Y/N / etoh, other substances Y/N / occupation:
FAM HX	ca / HTN / MI / CAD / stroke / hyperlipidemia / DM2 / Alzheimer's / depression / osteoporosis / other:

GENERAL	well appearing / well nourished / a&o x 3 / normal mood / normal affect
NEURO	intact / abnormal **DTR:** 1 2 3 4 5 location:
SKIN + NAILS	turgor / rash / bruising / lesions // texture, distribution of hair // nails: abnormal color / nail deformity
HEAD	normocephalic / atraumatic / visible mass / palpable mass / depression / scarring
EYES	acuity intact / conjunctiva clear / EOM intact / PERRLA / fundi: normal discs and vessels / icterus / exudate / hemorrhage
EARS	EACs clear / TM translucent, mobile / landmarks abnormal / hearing diminished
NOSE	lesions / mucosal inflammation / septum, turbinates abnormal / sinus tenderness
MOUTH	mucous membranes dry / lesions / poor dentition / caries / gingival inflammation
PHARYNX	mucosa inflammation / tonsillar hypertrophy / tonsillar exudate
NECK	supple / ROM WNL / lesion / bruit / adenopathy / thyroid enlarged, tender / mass
CARDIAC	regular rate, rhythm / S1, S2 / murmur / gallop / click / rub / PMI displacement
RESP	clear to auscultation in all fields / wheezes (insp) (exp) / rales / crackles
ABDOMEN	BSx4 / tender / organomegaly / mass / hernia
RECTAL	abnormal tone / hemorrhoids (int/ext) / palpable mass
BACK	abnormal curvature / tenderness / CVAT / Δ ROM
EXTREMITIES	amputation / deformity / edema / varicosities / + pulses
MSK	abnormal gait / asymmetry / crepitation / defect / tenderness / mass / effusion / Δ ROM / instability / atrophy / abnormal strength, tone in head, neck, spine, ribs, pelvis, UE, LE / pathologic reflexes
PSYCH	A&O x3 / +recent/remote memory / insight / affect
BREAST	nipple abnormality / mass / tenderness / axillary, clavicular adenopathy
GYN/GU	lesions / d/c / uterus, adnexa tenderness / CMT // circumcised / penile lesions / urethra normal location, no d/c / testes normal / + cremasteric reflex
FEET	+ pulses / monofilament + / nails abnormal / dry, broken skin / callus

LABS	CBC / CMP / lipids / TSH / microalbumin / A1C / UA, culture / PSA / iron studies / other:

DIAGNOSTICS	XR / MRI / CT / US / cardiac / other
REFERRALS	**F/U** ___ wk ___ mo

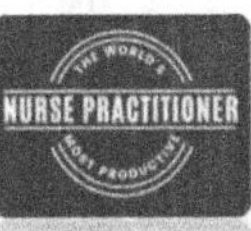

<table>
<tr><td colspan="2">

Patient ID#:   **Date of visit:**
Reason for visit: **Age:**   **Gender:**

</td><td>

BP: **HT:**
HR: **WT:**
T: **BMI:**
O2%:   **PAIN:**

NOTES . . . .

</td></tr>
</table>

CONST — Δ appetite, energy, weight / fever / chills / sweats / fatigue

HEAD — trauma / mass / tenderness / rash / lesions

EYES — visionΔ / itch / d/c / tears / dry / cataracts / glaucoma / glasses, contacts

ENT — hearing Δ / pain / d/c / vertigo / ? infection // epistaxis / congestion // bleeding, swelling gums / pain / sore throat / voice Δ // neck pain / lumps / swelling / difficulty swallowing

CARDIAC — pain / pressure / dizzy / N / orthopnea / edema / palp / weak w exertion / hx murmurs / hx MI / HTN / HF / numb / tingle / cold extrem / slow wound healing

RESP — wheeze / SOB / cough / asthma / bronch / COPD

GI — abd pain / Δ in bowels / constipation / diarrhea / N V / hepatitis / gallstones / dysphagia / reflux / hemorrhoids / black, bloody stools

GU — burn / pain / nocturia / polyuria / hematuria / incontinence / infection / kid. stones

GENITAL — DC / sores / pain / masses / last pap ______ / sexually active Y N / dyspareunia / LMP ______ / contraception

MSK — redness / swelling / warmth / pain / +/- ROM / arthritis / musc cramps / fracture / sprains / joint replacement / stiffness: AM PM

SKIN — rash / pruritis / jaundice / bruising / hx skin ca / mole Δ / Δ in hair, nails / lesions / slow wound healing

BREASTS — lump / pain / dc / last mammo ______ / self exams YN

NEURO — HA / seizure / vertigo / memory Δ / gait Δ / speech / coord

PSYCH — depression / anxiety / Δ in sleep pattern / substance, ETOH abuse / suicidal ideation / homicidal ideation

ENDO — polydipsia, polyuria / heat, cold intolerance / Δ hair/nails/energy

HEM/LYMPH — anemia / bruising / hx transfusions / blood disorder / lymphadenopathy / axillary, groin tenderness

ALLX/IMMUN — season allx / food allx / med allx / immune disorder:

SOCIAL HX — # in household ______ / lives with SP/BF/GF/SO / children __ / tobacco Y/N #pk / sexual activity Y/N / etoh, other substances Y/N / occupation:

FAM HX — ca / HTN / MI / CAD / stroke / hyperlipidemia / DM2 / Alzheimer's / depression / osteoporosis / other:

GENERAL — well appearing / well nourished / a&o x 3 / normal mood / normal affect

NEURO — intact / abnormal   **DTR:** 1 2 3 4 5 location:

SKIN + NAILS — turgor / rash / bruising / lesions // texture, distribution of hair // nails: abnormal color / nail deformity

HEAD — normocephalic / atraumatic / visible mass / palpable mass / depression / scarring

EYES — acuity intact / conjunctiva clear / EOM intact / PERRLA / fundi: normal discs and vessels / icterus / exudate / hemorrhage

EARS — EACs clear / TM translucent, mobile / landmarks abnormal / hearing diminished

NOSE — lesions / mucosal inflammation / septum, turbinates abnormal / sinus tenderness

MOUTH — mucous membranes dry / lesions / poor dentition / caries / gingival inflammation

PHARYNX — mucosa inflammation / tonsillar hypertrophy / tonsillar exudate

NECK — supple / ROM WNL / lesion / bruit / adenopathy / thyroid enlarged, tender / mass

CARDIAC — regular rate, rhythm / S1, S2 / murmur / gallop / click / rub / PMI displacement

RESP — clear to auscultation in all fields / wheezes (insp) (exp) / rales / crackles

ABDOMEN — BSx4 / tender / organomegaly / mass / hernia

RECTAL — abnormal tone / hemorrhoids (int/ext) / palpable mass

BACK — abnormal curvature / tenderness / CVAT / Δ ROM

EXTREMITIES — amputation / deformity / edema / varicosities / + pulses

MSK — abnormal gait / asymmetry / crepitation / defect / tenderness / mass / effusion / Δ ROM / instability / atrophy / abnormal strength, tone in head, neck, spine, ribs, pelvis, UE, LE / pathologic reflexes

PSYCH — A&O x3 / +recent/remote memory / insight / affect

BREAST — nipple abnormality / mass / tenderness / axillary, clavicular adenopathy

GYN/GU — lesions / d/c / uterus, adnexa tenderness / CMT // circumcised / penile lesions / urethra normal location, no d/c / testes normal / + cremasteric reflex

FEET — + pulses / monofilament + / nails abnormal / dry, broken skin / callus

---

LABS — CBC / CMP / lipids / TSH / microalbumin / A1C / UA, culture / PSA / iron studies / other:

DIAGNOSTICS — XR / MRI / CT / US / cardiac / other

REFERRALS —   **F/U** ___ wk ___ mo

<table>
<tr><td colspan="2">Patient ID#:
Reason for visit:</td><td>Date of visit:
Age: Gender:</td></tr>
</table>

BP: HT:
HR: WT:
T: BMI:
O2%:   PAIN:

NOTES . . . .

CONST	Δ appetite, energy, weight / fever / chills / sweats / fatigue
HEAD	trauma / mass / tenderness / rash / lesions
EYES	visionΔ / itch / d/c / tears / dry / cataracts / glaucoma / glasses, contacts
ENT	hearing Δ / pain / d/c / vertigo / ? infection // epistaxis / congestion // bleeding, swelling gums / pain / sore throat / voice Δ // neck pain / lumps / swelling / difficulty swallowing
CARDIAC	pain / pressure / dizzy / N / orthopnea / edema / palp / weak w exertion / hx murmurs / hx MI / HTN / HF / numb / tingle / cold extrem / slow wound healing
RESP	wheeze / SOB / cough / asthma / bronch / COPD
GI	abd pain / Δ in bowels / constipation / diarrhea / N V / hepatitis / gallstones / dysphagia / reflux / hemorrhoids / black, bloody stools
GU	burn / pain / nocturia / polyuria / hematuria / incontinence / infection / kid. stones
GENITAL	DC / sores / pain / masses / last pap _____ / sexually active Y N / dyspareunia / LMP _____ / contraception
MSK	redness / swelling / warmth / pain / +/- ROM / arthritis / musc cramps / fracture / sprains / joint replacement / stiffness: AM PM
SKIN	rash / pruritis / jaundice / bruising / hx skin ca / mole Δ / Δ in hair, nails / lesions / slow wound healing
BREASTS	lump / pain / dc / last mammo _____ / self exams YN
NEURO	HA / seizure / vertigo / memory Δ / gait Δ / speech / coord
PSYCH	depression / anxiety / Δ in sleep pattern / substance, ETOH abuse / suicidal ideation / homicidal ideation
ENDO	polydipsia, polyuria / heat, cold intolerance / Δ hair/nails/energy
HEM/LYMPH	anemia / bruising / hx transfusions / blood disorder / lymphadenopathy / axillary, groin tenderness
ALLX/IMMUN	season allx / food allx / med allx / immune disorder:

SOCIAL HX	# in household _____ / lives with SP/BF/GF/SO / children __ / tobacco Y/N #pk / sexual activity Y/N / etoh, other substances Y/N / occupation:
FAM HX	ca / HTN / MI / CAD / stroke / hyperlipidemia / DM2 / Alzheimer's / depression / osteoporosis / other:

GENERAL	well appearing / well nourished / a&o x 3 / normal mood / normal affect
NEURO	intact / abnormal **DTR:** 1 2 3 4 5 location:
SKIN + NAILS	turgor / rash / bruising / lesions // texture, distribution of hair // nails: abnormal color / nail deformity
HEAD	normocephalic / atraumatic / visible mass / palpable mass / depression / scarring
EYES	acuity intact / conjunctiva clear / EOM intact / PERRLA / fundi: normal discs and vessels / icterus / exudate / hemorrhage
EARS	EACs clear / TM translucent, mobile / landmarks abnormal / hearing diminished
NOSE	lesions / mucosal inflammation / septum, turbinates abnormal / sinus tenderness
MOUTH	mucous membranes dry / lesions / poor dentition / caries / gingival inflammation
PHARYNX	mucosa inflammation / tonsillar hypertrophy / tonsillar exudate
NECK	supple / ROM WNL / lesion / bruit / adenopathy / thyroid enlarged, tender / mass
CARDIAC	regular rate, rhythm / S1, S2 / murmur / gallop / click / rub / PMI displacement
RESP	clear to auscultation in all fields / wheezes (insp) (exp) / rales / crackles
ABDOMEN	BSx4 / tender / organomegaly / mass / hernia
RECTAL	abnormal tone / hemorrhoids (int/ext) / palpable mass
BACK	abnormal curvature / tenderness / CVAT / Δ ROM
EXTREMITIES	amputation / deformity / edema / varicosities / + pulses
MSK	abnormal gait / asymmetry / crepitation / defect / tenderness / mass / effusion / Δ ROM / instability / atrophy / abnormal strength, tone in head, neck, spine, ribs, pelvis, UE, LE / pathologic reflexes
PSYCH	A&O x3 / +recent/remote memory / insight / affect
BREAST	nipple abnormality / mass / tenderness / axillary, clavicular adenopathy
GYN/GU	lesions / d/c / uterus, adnexa tenderness / CMT // circumcised / penile lesions / urethra normal location, no d/c / testes normal / + cremasteric reflex
FEET	+ pulses / monofilament + / nails abnormal / dry, broken skin / callus

LABS	CBC / CMP / lipids / TSH / microalbumin / A1C / UA, culture / PSA / iron studies / other:

DIAGNOSTICS	XR / MRI / CT / US / cardiac / other
REFERRALS	**F/U** ___ wk ___ mo

| Patient ID#: | Date of visit: |
| Reason for visit: | Age: Gender: |

BP: HT:
HR: WT:
T: BMI:
O2%:   PAIN:

NOTES . . . .

CONST Δ appetite, energy, weight / fever / chills / sweats / fatigue
HEAD trauma / mass / tenderness / rash / lesions
EYES visionΔ / itch / d/c / tears / dry / cataracts / glaucoma / glasses, contacts
ENT hearing Δ / pain / d/c / vertigo / ? infection // epistaxis / congestion // bleeding, swelling gums / pain / sore throat / voice Δ // neck pain / lumps / swelling / difficulty swallowing
CARDIAC pain / pressure / dizzy / N / orthopnea / edema / palp / weak w exertion / hx murmurs / hx MI / HTN / HF / numb / tingle / cold extrem / slow wound healing
RESP wheeze / SOB / cough / asthma / bronch / COPD
GI abd pain / Δ in bowels / constipation / diarrhea / N V / hepatitis / gallstones / dysphagia / reflux / hemorrhoids / black, bloody stools
GU burn / pain / nocturia / polyuria / hematuria / incontinence / infection / kid. stones
GENITAL DC / sores / pain / masses / last pap _____ / sexually active Y N / dyspareunia / LMP _______ / contraception
MSK redness / swelling / warmth / pain / +/- ROM / arthritis / musc cramps / fracture / sprains / joint replacement / stiffness: AM PM
SKIN rash / pruritis / jaundice / bruising / hx skin ca / mole Δ / Δ in hair, nails / lesions / slow wound healing
BREASTS lump / pain / dc / last mammo _______ / self exams YN
NEURO HA / seizure / vertigo / memory Δ / gait Δ / speech / coord
PSYCH depression / anxiety / Δ in sleep pattern / substance, ETOH abuse / suicidal ideation / homicidal ideation
ENDO polydipsia, polyuria / heat, cold intolerance / Δ hair/nails/energy
HEM/LYMPH anemia / bruising / hx transfusions / blood disorder / lymphadenopathy / axillary, groin tenderness
ALLX/IMMUN season allx / food allx / med allx / immune disorder:

SOCIAL HX # in household _______ / lives with SP/BF/GF/SO / children ___ / tobacco Y/N #pk / sexual activity Y/N / etoh, other substances Y/N / occupation:
FAM HX ca / HTN / MI / CAD / stroke / hyperlipidemia / DM2 / Alzheimer's / depression / osteoporosis / other:

GENERAL well appearing / well nourished / a&o x 3 / normal mood / normal affect
NEURO intact / abnormal   **DTR:** 1 2 3 4 5 location:
SKIN + NAILS turgor / rash / bruising / lesions // texture, distribution of hair // nails: abnormal color / nail deformity
HEAD normocephalic / atraumatic / visible mass / palpable mass / depression / scarring
EYES acuity intact / conjunctiva clear / EOM intact / PERRLA / fundi: normal discs and vessels / icterus / exudate / hemorrhage
EARS EACs clear / TM translucent, mobile / landmarks abnormal / hearing diminished
NOSE lesions / mucosal inflammation / septum, turbinates abnormal / sinus tenderness
MOUTH mucous membranes dry / lesions / poor dentition / caries / gingival inflammation
PHARYNX mucosa inflammation / tonsillar hypertrophy / tonsillar exudate
NECK supple / ROM WNL / lesion / bruit / adenopathy / thyroid enlarged, tender / mass
CARDIAC regular rate, rhythm / S1, S2 / murmur / gallop / click / rub / PMI displacement
RESP clear to auscultation in all fields / wheezes (insp) (exp) / rales / crackles
ABDOMEN BSx4 / tender / organomegaly / mass / hernia
RECTAL abnormal tone / hemorrhoids (int/ext) / palpable mass
BACK abnormal curvature / tenderness / CVAT / Δ ROM
EXTREMITIES amputation / deformity / edema / varicosities / + pulses
MSK abnormal gait / asymmetry / crepitation / defect / tenderness / mass / effusion / Δ ROM / instability / atrophy / abnormal strength, tone in head, neck, spine, ribs, pelvis, UE, LE / pathologic reflexes
PSYCH A&O x3 / +recent/remote memory / insight / affect
BREAST nipple abnormality / mass / tenderness / axillary, clavicular adenopathy
GYN/GU lesions / d/c / uterus, adnexa tenderness / CMT // circumcised / penile lesions / urethra normal location, no d/c / testes normal / + cremasteric reflex
FEET + pulses / monofilament + / nails abnormal / dry, broken skin / callus

LABS CBC / CMP / lipids / TSH / microalbumin / A1C / UA, culture / PSA / iron studies / other:

DIAGNOSTICS XR / MRI / CT / US / cardiac / other
REFERRALS   **F/U** ___ wk ___ mo

<table>
<tr><td>

Patient ID#:   **Date of visit:**

Reason for visit: **Age:**   **Gender:**

</td><td>

BP: **HT:**
HR: **WT:**
T: **BMI:**
O2%:   **PAIN:**

NOTES . . . .

</td></tr>
</table>

CONST — Δ appetite, energy, weight / fever / chills / sweats / fatigue

HEAD — trauma / mass / tenderness / rash / lesions

EYES — visionΔ / itch / d/c / tears / dry / cataracts / glaucoma / glasses, contacts

ENT — hearing Δ / pain / d/c / vertigo / ? infection // epistaxis / congestion // bleeding, swelling gums / pain / sore throat / voice Δ // neck pain / lumps / swelling / difficulty swallowing

CARDIAC — pain / pressure / dizzy / N / orthopnea / edema / palp / weak w exertion / hx murmurs / hx MI / HTN / HF / numb / tingle / cold extrem / slow wound healing

RESP — wheeze / SOB / cough / asthma / bronch / COPD

GI — abd pain / Δ in bowels / constipation / diarrhea / N V / hepatitis / gallstones / dysphagia / reflux / hemorrhoids / black, bloody stools

GU — burn / pain / nocturia / polyuria / hematuria / incontinence / infection / kid. stones

GENITAL — DC / sores / pain / masses / last pap _____ / sexually active Y N / dyspareunia / LMP _______ / contraception

MSK — redness / swelling / warmth / pain / +/- ROM / arthritis / musc cramps / fracture / sprains / joint replacement / stiffness: AM PM

SKIN — rash / pruritis / jaundice / bruising / hx skin ca / mole Δ / Δ in hair, nails / lesions / slow wound healing

BREASTS — lump / pain / dc / last mammo _______ / self exams YN

NEURO — HA / seizure / vertigo / memory Δ / gait Δ / speech / coord

PSYCH — depression / anxiety / Δ in sleep pattern / substance, ETOH abuse / suicidal ideation / homicidal ideation

ENDO — polydipsia, polyuria / heat, cold intolerance / Δ hair/nails/energy

HEM/LYMPH — anemia / bruising / hx transfusions / blood disorder / lymphadenopathy / axillary, groin tenderness

ALLX/IMMUN — season allx / food allx / med allx / immune disorder:

SOCIAL HX — # in household _____ / lives with SP/BF/GF/SO / children __ / tobacco Y/N #pk / sexual activity Y/N / etoh, other substances Y/N / occupation:

FAM HX — ca / HTN / MI / CAD / stroke / hyperlipidemia / DM2 / Alzheimer's / depression / osteoporosis / other:

GENERAL — well appearing / well nourished / a&o x 3 / normal mood / normal affect

NEURO — intact / abnormal   **DTR:** 1 2 3 4 5 location:

SKIN + NAILS — turgor / rash / bruising / lesions // texture, distribution of hair // nails: abnormal color / nail deformity

HEAD — normocephalic / atraumatic / visible mass / palpable mass / depression / scarring

EYES — acuity intact / conjunctiva clear / EOM intact / PERRLA / fundi: normal discs and vessels / icterus / exudate / hemorrhage

EARS — EACs clear / TM translucent, mobile / landmarks abnormal / hearing diminished

NOSE — lesions / mucosal inflammation / septum, turbinates abnormal / sinus tenderness

MOUTH — mucous membranes dry / lesions / poor dentition / caries / gingival inflammation

PHARYNX — mucosa inflammation / tonsillar hypertrophy / tonsillar exudate

NECK — supple / ROM WNL / lesion / bruit / adenopathy / thyroid enlarged, tender / mass

CARDIAC — regular rate, rhythm / S1, S2 / murmur / gallop / click / rub / PMI displacement

RESP — clear to auscultation in all fields / wheezes (insp) (exp) / rales / crackles

ABDOMEN — BSx4 / tender / organomegaly / mass / hernia

RECTAL — abnormal tone / hemorrhoids (int/ext) / palpable mass

BACK — abnormal curvature / tenderness / CVAT / Δ ROM

EXTREMITIES — amputation / deformity / edema / varicosities / + pulses

MSK — abnormal gait / asymmetry / crepitation / defect / tenderness / mass / effusion / Δ ROM / instability / atrophy / abnormal strength, tone in head, neck, spine, ribs, pelvis, UE, LE / pathologic reflexes

PSYCH — A&O x3 / +recent/remote memory / insight / affect

BREAST — nipple abnormality / mass / tenderness / axillary, clavicular adenopathy

GYN/GU — lesions / d/c / uterus, adnexa tenderness / CMT // circumcised / penile lesions / urethra normal location, no d/c / testes normal / + cremasteric reflex

FEET — + pulses / monofilament + / nails abnormal / dry, broken skin / callus

---

LABS — CBC / CMP / lipids / TSH / microalbumin / A1C / UA, culture / PSA / iron studies / other:

DIAGNOSTICS — XR / MRI / CT / US / cardiac / other

REFERRALS —   **F/U** ___ wk ___ mo

<table>
<tr><td colspan="2">

Patient ID#:
Reason for visit:

</td><td>

Date of visit:
Age: **Gender:**

</td></tr>
</table>

BP:	HT:
HR:	WT:
T:	BMI:
O2%:	PAIN:

NOTES . . . .

CONST	Δ appetite, energy, weight / fever / chills / sweats / fatigue
HEAD	trauma / mass / tenderness / rash / lesions
EYES	visionΔ / itch / d/c / tears / dry / cataracts / glaucoma / glasses, contacts
ENT	hearing Δ / pain / d/c / vertigo / ? infection // epistaxis / congestion // bleeding, swelling gums / pain / sore throat / voice Δ // neck pain / lumps / swelling / difficulty swallowing
CARDIAC	pain / pressure / dizzy / N / orthopnea / edema / palp / weak w exertion / hx murmurs / hx MI / HTN / HF / numb / tingle / cold extrem / slow wound healing
RESP	wheeze / SOB / cough / asthma / bronch / COPD
GI	abd pain / Δ in bowels / constipation / diarrhea / N V / hepatitis / gallstones / dysphagia / reflux / hemorrhoids / black, bloody stools
GU	burn / pain / nocturia / polyuria / hematuria / incontinence / infection / kid. stones
GENITAL	DC / sores / pain / masses / last pap ______ / sexually active Y N / dyspareunia / LMP ______ / contraception
MSK	redness / swelling / warmth / pain / +/- ROM / arthritis / musc cramps / fracture / sprains / joint replacement / stiffness: AM PM
SKIN	rash / pruritis / jaundice / bruising / hx skin ca / mole Δ / Δ in hair, nails / lesions / slow wound healing
BREASTS	lump / pain / dc / last mammo ______ / self exams YN
NEURO	HA / seizure / vertigo / memory Δ / gait Δ / speech / coord
PSYCH	depression / anxiety / Δ in sleep pattern / substance, ETOH abuse / suicidal ideation / homicidal ideation
ENDO	polydipsia, polyuria / heat, cold intolerance / Δ hair/nails/energy
HEM/LYMPH	anemia / bruising / hx transfusions / blood disorder / lymphadenopathy / axillary, groin tenderness
ALLX/IMMUN	season allx / food allx / med allx / immune disorder:

SOCIAL HX	# in household ______ / lives with SP/BF/GF/SO / children __ / tobacco Y/N #pk / sexual activity Y/N / etoh, other substances Y/N / occupation:
FAM HX	ca / HTN / MI / CAD / stroke / hyperlipidemia / DM2 / Alzheimer's / depression / osteoporosis / other:

GENERAL	well appearing / well nourished / a&o x 3 / normal mood / normal affect
NEURO	intact / abnormal **DTR:** 1 2 3 4 5 location:
SKIN + NAILS	turgor / rash / bruising / lesions // texture, distribution of hair // nails: abnormal color / nail deformity
HEAD	normocephalic / atraumatic / visible mass / palpable mass / depression / scarring
EYES	acuity intact / conjunctiva clear / EOM intact / PERRLA / fundi: normal discs and vessels / icterus / exudate / hemorrhage
EARS	EACs clear / TM translucent, mobile / landmarks abnormal / hearing diminished
NOSE	lesions / mucosal inflammation / septum, turbinates abnormal / sinus tenderness
MOUTH	mucous membranes dry / lesions / poor dentition / caries / gingival inflammation
PHARYNX	mucosa inflammation / tonsillar hypertrophy / tonsillar exudate
NECK	supple / ROM WNL / lesion / bruit / adenopathy / thyroid enlarged, tender / mass
CARDIAC	regular rate, rhythm / S1, S2 / murmur / gallop / click / rub / PMI displacement
RESP	clear to auscultation in all fields / wheezes (insp) (exp) / rales / crackles
ABDOMEN	BSx4 / tender / organomegaly / mass / hernia
RECTAL	abnormal tone / hemorrhoids (int/ext) / palpable mass
BACK	abnormal curvature / tenderness / CVAT / Δ ROM
EXTREMITIES	amputation / deformity / edema / varicosities / + pulses
MSK	abnormal gait / asymmetry / crepitation / defect / tenderness / mass / effusion / Δ ROM / instability / atrophy / abnormal strength, tone in head, neck, spine, ribs, pelvis, UE, LE / pathologic reflexes
PSYCH	A&O x3 / +recent/remote memory / insight / affect
BREAST	nipple abnormality / mass / tenderness / axillary, clavicular adenopathy
GYN/GU	lesions / d/c / uterus, adnexa tenderness / CMT // circumcised / penile lesions / urethra normal location, no d/c / testes normal / + cremasteric reflex
FEET	+ pulses / monofilament + / nails abnormal / dry, broken skin / callus

LABS	CBC / CMP / lipids / TSH / microalbumin / A1C / UA, culture / PSA / iron studies / other:

DIAGNOSTICS	XR / MRI / CT / US / cardiac / other
REFERRALS	**F/U** ___ wk ___ mo

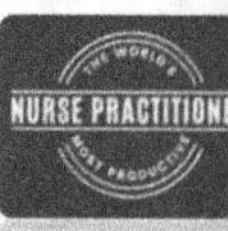

<table>
<tr><td colspan="2">Patient ID#:</td><td>Date of visit:</td></tr>
<tr><td colspan="2">Reason for visit:</td><td>Age: Gender:</td></tr>
</table>

BP:	**HT:**
HR:	**WT:**
T:	**BMI:**
O2%:	**PAIN:**

NOTES . . . .

CONST	Δ appetite, energy, weight / fever / chills / sweats / fatigue
HEAD	trauma / mass / tenderness / rash / lesions
EYES	visionΔ / itch / d/c / tears / dry / cataracts / glaucoma / glasses, contacts
ENT	hearing Δ / pain / d/c / vertigo / ? infection // epistaxis / congestion // bleeding, swelling gums / pain / sore throat / voice Δ // neck pain / lumps / swelling / difficulty swallowing
CARDIAC	pain / pressure / dizzy / N / orthopnea / edema / palp / weak w exertion / hx murmurs / hx MI / HTN / HF / numb / tingle / cold extrem / slow wound healing
RESP	wheeze / SOB / cough / asthma / bronch / COPD
GI	abd pain / Δ in bowels / constipation / diarrhea / N V / hepatitis / gallstones / dysphagia / reflux / hemorrhoids / black, bloody stools
GU	burn / pain / nocturia / polyuria / hematuria / incontinence / infection / kid. stones
GENITAL	DC / sores / pain / masses / last pap _____ / sexually active Y N / dyspareunia / LMP _______ / contraception
MSK	redness / swelling / warmth / pain / +/- ROM / arthritis / musc cramps / fracture / sprains / joint replacement / stiffness: AM PM
SKIN	rash / pruritis / jaundice / bruising / hx skin ca / mole Δ / Δ in hair, nails / lesions / slow wound healing
BREASTS	lump / pain / dc / last mammo _______ / self exams YN
NEURO	HA / seizure / vertigo / memory Δ / gait Δ / speech / coord
PSYCH	depression / anxiety / Δ in sleep pattern / substance, ETOH abuse / suicidal ideation / homicidal ideation
ENDO	polydipsia, polyuria / heat, cold intolerance / Δ hair/nails/energy
HEM/LYMPH	anemia / bruising / hx transfusions / blood disorder / lymphadenopathy / axillary, groin tenderness
ALLX/IMMUN	season allx / food allx / med allx / immune disorder:

SOCIAL HX	# in household _____ / lives with SP/BF/GF/SO / children __ / tobacco Y/N #pk / sexual activity Y/N / etoh, other substances Y/N / occupation:
FAM HX	ca / HTN / MI / CAD / stroke / hyperlipidemia / DM2 / Alzheimer's / depression / osteoporosis / other:

GENERAL	well appearing / well nourished / a&o x 3 / normal mood / normal affect
NEURO	intact / abnormal **DTR:** 1 2 3 4 5 location:
SKIN + NAILS	turgor / rash / bruising / lesions // texture, distribution of hair // nails: abnormal color / nail deformity
HEAD	normocephalic / atraumatic / visible mass / palpable mass / depression / scarring
EYES	acuity intact / conjunctiva clear / EOM intact / PERRLA / fundi: normal discs and vessels / icterus / exudate / hemorrhage
EARS	EACs clear / TM translucent, mobile / landmarks abnormal / hearing diminished
NOSE	lesions / mucosal inflammation / septum, turbinates abnormal / sinus tenderness
MOUTH	mucous membranes dry / lesions / poor dentition / caries / gingival inflammation
PHARYNX	mucosa inflammation / tonsillar hypertrophy / tonsillar exudate
NECK	supple / ROM WNL / lesion / bruit / adenopathy / thyroid enlarged, tender / mass
CARDIAC	regular rate, rhythm / S1, S2 / murmur / gallop / click / rub / PMI displacement
RESP	clear to auscultation in all fields / wheezes (insp) (exp) / rales / crackles
ABDOMEN	BSx4 / tender / organomegaly / mass / hernia
RECTAL	abnormal tone / hemorrhoids (int/ext) / palpable mass
BACK	abnormal curvature / tenderness / CVAT / Δ ROM
EXTREMITIES	amputation / deformity / edema / varicosities / + pulses
MSK	abnormal gait / asymmetry / crepitation / defect / tenderness / mass / effusion / Δ ROM / instability / atrophy / abnormal strength, tone in head, neck, spine, ribs, pelvis, UE, LE / pathologic reflexes
PSYCH	A&O x3 / +recent/remote memory / insight / affect
BREAST	nipple abnormality / mass / tenderness / axillary, clavicular adenopathy
GYN/GU	lesions / d/c / uterus, adnexa tenderness / CMT // circumcised / penile lesions / urethra normal location, no d/c / testes normal / + cremasteric reflex
FEET	+ pulses / monofilament + / nails abnormal / dry, broken skin / callus

LABS	CBC / CMP / lipids / TSH / microalbumin / A1C / UA, culture / PSA / iron studies / other:

DIAGNOSTICS	XR / MRI / CT / US / cardiac / other
REFERRALS	**F/U** ___ wk ___ mo

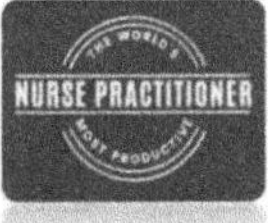

Patient ID#:	Date of visit:
Reason for visit:	Age: Gender:

BP: **HT:**
HR: **WT:**
T: **BMI:**
O2%:   **PAIN:**

NOTES . . . .

CONST	Δ appetite, energy, weight / fever / chills / sweats / fatigue
HEAD	trauma / mass / tenderness / rash / lesions
EYES	visionΔ / itch / d/c / tears / dry / cataracts / glaucoma / glasses, contacts
ENT	hearing Δ / pain / d/c / vertigo / ? infection // epistaxis / congestion // bleeding, swelling gums / pain / sore throat / voice Δ // neck pain / lumps / swelling / difficulty swallowing
CARDIAC	pain / pressure / dizzy / N / orthopnea / edema / palp / weak w exertion / hx murmurs / hx MI / HTN / HF / numb / tingle / cold extrem / slow wound healing
RESP	wheeze / SOB / cough / asthma / bronch / COPD
GI	abd pain / Δ in bowels / constipation / diarrhea / N V / hepatitis / gallstones / dysphagia / reflux / hemorrhoids / black, bloody stools
GU	burn / pain / nocturia / polyuria / hematuria / incontinence / infection / kid. stones
GENITAL	DC / sores / pain / masses / last pap ______ / sexually active Y N / dyspareunia / LMP ______ / contraception
MSK	redness / swelling / warmth / pain / +/- ROM / arthritis / musc cramps / fracture / sprains / joint replacement / stiffness: AM PM
SKIN	rash / pruritis / jaundice / bruising / hx skin ca / mole Δ / Δ in hair, nails / lesions / slow wound healing
BREASTS	lump / pain / dc / last mammo ______ / self exams YN
NEURO	HA / seizure / vertigo / memory Δ / gait Δ / speech / coord
PSYCH	depression / anxiety / Δ in sleep pattern / substance, ETOH abuse / suicidal ideation / homicidal ideation
ENDO	polydipsia, polyuria / heat, cold intolerance / Δ hair/nails/energy
HEM/LYMPH	anemia / bruising / hx transfusions / blood disorder / lymphadenopathy / axillary, groin tenderness
ALLX/IMMUN	season allx / food allx / med allx / immune disorder:

SOCIAL HX	# in household ______ / lives with SP/BF/GF/SO / children __ / tobacco Y/N #pk / sexual activity Y/N / etoh, other substances Y/N / occupation:
FAM HX	ca / HTN / MI / CAD / stroke / hyperlipidemia / DM2 / Alzheimer's / depression / osteoporosis / other:

GENERAL	well appearing / well nourished / a&o x 3 / normal mood / normal affect
NEURO	intact / abnormal **DTR:** 1 2 3 4 5 location:
SKIN + NAILS	turgor / rash / bruising / lesions // texture, distribution of hair // nails: abnormal color / nail deformity
HEAD	normocephalic / atraumatic / visible mass / palpable mass / depression / scarring
EYES	acuity intact / conjunctiva clear / EOM intact / PERRLA / fundi: normal discs and vessels / icterus / exudate / hemorrhage
EARS	EACs clear / TM translucent, mobile / landmarks abnormal / hearing diminished
NOSE	lesions / mucosal inflammation / septum, turbinates abnormal / sinus tenderness
MOUTH	mucous membranes dry / lesions / poor dentition / caries / gingival inflammation
PHARYNX	mucosa inflammation / tonsillar hypertrophy / tonsillar exudate
NECK	supple / ROM WNL / lesion / bruit / adenopathy / thyroid enlarged, tender / mass
CARDIAC	regular rate, rhythm / S1, S2 / murmur / gallop / click / rub / PMI displacement
RESP	clear to auscultation in all fields / wheezes (insp) (exp) / rales / crackles
ABDOMEN	BSx4 / tender / organomegaly / mass / hernia
RECTAL	abnormal tone / hemorrhoids (int/ext) / palpable mass
BACK	abnormal curvature / tenderness / CVAT / Δ ROM
EXTREMITIES	amputation / deformity / edema / varicosities / + pulses
MSK	abnormal gait / asymmetry / crepitation / defect / tenderness / mass / effusion / Δ ROM / instability / atrophy / abnormal strength, tone in head, neck, spine, ribs, pelvis, UE, LE / pathologic reflexes
PSYCH	A&O x3 / +recent/remote memory / insight / affect
BREAST	nipple abnormality / mass / tenderness / axillary, clavicular adenopathy
GYN/GU	lesions / d/c / uterus, adnexa tenderness / CMT // circumcised / penile lesions / urethra normal location, no d/c / testes normal / + cremasteric reflex
FEET	+ pulses / monofilament + / nails abnormal / dry, broken skin / callus

LABS	CBC / CMP / lipids / TSH / microalbumin / A1C / UA, culture / PSA / iron studies / other:

DIAGNOSTICS	XR / MRI / CT / US / cardiac / other
REFERRALS	**F/U** ___ wk ___ mo

<table>
<tr><td>Patient ID#:</td><td>Date of visit:</td></tr>
<tr><td>Reason for visit:</td><td>Age: Gender:</td></tr>
</table>

BP: **HT:**
HR: **WT:**
T: **BMI:**
O2%:   **PAIN:**

NOTES . . . .

CONST	Δ appetite, energy, weight / fever / chills / sweats / fatigue
HEAD	trauma / mass / tenderness / rash / lesions
EYES	visionΔ / itch / d/c / tears / dry / cataracts / glaucoma / glasses, contacts
ENT	hearing Δ / pain / d/c / vertigo / ? infection **//** epistaxis / congestion **//** bleeding, swelling gums / pain / sore throat / voice Δ **//** neck pain / lumps / swelling / difficulty swallowing
CARDIAC	pain / pressure / dizzy / N / orthopnea / edema / palp / weak w exertion / hx murmurs / hx MI / HTN / HF / numb / tingle / cold extrem / slow wound healing
RESP	wheeze / SOB / cough / asthma / bronch / COPD
GI	abd pain / Δ in bowels / constipation / diarrhea / N V / hepatitis / gallstones / dysphagia / reflux / hemorrhoids / black, bloody stools
GU	burn / pain / nocturia / polyuria / hematuria / incontinence / infection / kid. stones
GENITAL	DC / sores / pain / masses / last pap _____ / sexually active Y N / dyspareunia / LMP _____ / contraception
MSK	redness / swelling / warmth / pain / +/- ROM / arthritis / musc cramps / fracture / sprains / joint replacement / stiffness: AM PM
SKIN	rash / pruritis / jaundice / bruising / hx skin ca / mole Δ / Δ in hair, nails / lesions / slow wound healing
BREASTS	lump / pain / dc / last mammo _____ / self exams YN
NEURO	HA / seizure / vertigo / memory Δ / gait Δ / speech / coord
PSYCH	depression / anxiety / Δ in sleep pattern / substance, ETOH abuse / suicidal ideation / homicidal ideation
ENDO	polydipsia, polyuria / heat, cold intolerance / Δ hair/nails/energy
HEM/LYMPH	anemia / bruising / hx transfusions / blood disorder / lymphadenopathy / axillary, groin tenderness
ALLX/IMMUN	season allx / food allx / med allx / immune disorder:
SOCIAL HX	# in household _____ / lives with SP/BF/GF/SO / children __ / tobacco Y/N #pk / sexual activity Y/N / etoh, other substances Y/N / occupation:
FAM HX	ca / HTN / MI / CAD / stroke / hyperlipidemia / DM2 / Alzheimer's / depression / osteoporosis / other:
GENERAL	well appearing / well nourished / a&o x 3 / normal mood / normal affect
NEURO	intact / abnormal **DTR:** 1 2 3 4 5 location:
SKIN + NAILS	turgor / rash / bruising / lesions **//** texture, distribution of hair **//** nails: abnormal color / nail deformity
HEAD	normocephalic / atraumatic / visible mass / palpable mass / depression / scarring
EYES	acuity intact / conjunctiva clear / EOM intact / PERRLA / fundi: normal discs and vessels / icterus / exudate / hemorrhage
EARS	EACs clear / TM translucent, mobile / landmarks abnormal / hearing diminished
NOSE	lesions / mucosal inflammation / septum, turbinates abnormal / sinus tenderness
MOUTH	mucous membranes dry / lesions / poor dentition / caries / gingival inflammation
PHARYNX	mucosa inflammation / tonsillar hypertrophy / tonsillar exudate
NECK	supple / ROM WNL / lesion / bruit / adenopathy / thyroid enlarged, tender / mass
CARDIAC	regular rate, rhythm / S1, S2 / murmur / gallop / click / rub / PMI displacement
RESP	clear to auscultation in all fields / wheezes (insp) (exp) / rales / crackles
ABDOMEN	BSx4 / tender / organomegaly / mass / hernia
RECTAL	abnormal tone / hemorrhoids (int/ext) / palpable mass
BACK	abnormal curvature / tenderness / CVAT / Δ ROM
EXTREMITIES	amputation / deformity / edema / varicosities / + pulses
MSK	abnormal gait / asymmetry / crepitation / defect / tenderness / mass / effusion / Δ ROM / instability / atrophy / abnormal strength, tone in head, neck, spine, ribs, pelvis, UE, LE / pathologic reflexes
PSYCH	A&O x3 / +recent/remote memory / insight / affect
BREAST	nipple abnormality / mass / tenderness / axillary, clavicular adenopathy
GYN/GU	lesions / d/c / uterus, adnexa tenderness / CMT **//** circumcised / penile lesions / urethra normal location, no d/c / testes normal / + cremasteric reflex
FEET	+ pulses / monofilament + / nails abnormal / dry, broken skin / callus
LABS	CBC / CMP / lipids / TSH / microalbumin / A1C / UA, culture / PSA / iron studies / other:
DIAGNOSTICS	XR / MRI / CT / US / cardiac / other
REFERRALS	**F/U** ___ wk ___ mo

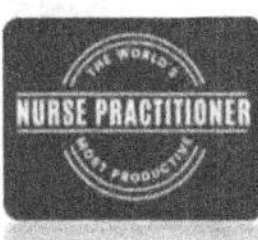

<table>
<tr><td colspan="2">Patient ID#:
Reason for visit:</td><td>Date of visit:
Age: Gender:</td></tr>
</table>

BP: HT:
HR: WT:
T: BMI:
O2%:   PAIN:

NOTES . . . .

CONST	Δ appetite, energy, weight / fever / chills / sweats / fatigue
HEAD	trauma / mass / tenderness / rash / lesions
EYES	visionΔ / itch / d/c / tears / dry / cataracts / glaucoma / glasses, contacts
ENT	hearing Δ / pain / d/c / vertigo / ? infection // epistaxis / congestion // bleeding, swelling gums / pain / sore throat / voice Δ // neck pain / lumps / swelling / difficulty swallowing
CARDIAC	pain / pressure / dizzy / N / orthopnea / edema / palp / weak w exertion / hx murmurs / hx MI / HTN / HF / numb / tingle / cold extrem / slow wound healing
RESP	wheeze / SOB / cough / asthma / bronch / COPD
GI	abd pain / Δ in bowels / constipation / diarrhea / N V / hepatitis / gallstones / dysphagia / reflux / hemorrhoids / black, bloody stools
GU	burn / pain / nocturia / polyuria / hematuria / incontinence / infection / kid. stones
GENITAL	DC / sores / pain / masses / last pap _____ / sexually active Y N / dyspareunia / LMP ______ / contraception
MSK	redness / swelling / warmth / pain / +/- ROM / arthritis / musc cramps / fracture / sprains / joint replacement / stiffness: AM PM
SKIN	rash / pruritis / jaundice / bruising / hx skin ca / mole Δ / Δ in hair, nails / lesions / slow wound healing
BREASTS	lump / pain / dc / last mammo ______ / self exams YN
NEURO	HA / seizure / vertigo / memory Δ / gait Δ / speech / coord
PSYCH	depression / anxiety / Δ in sleep pattern / substance, ETOH abuse / suicidal ideation / homicidal ideation
ENDO	polydipsia, polyuria / heat, cold intolerance / Δ hair/nails/energy
HEM/LYMPH	anemia / bruising / hx transfusions / blood disorder / lymphadenopathy / axillary, groin tenderness
ALLX/IMMUN	season allx / food allx / med allx / immune disorder:

SOCIAL HX	# in household ______ / lives with SP/BF/GF/SO / children __ / tobacco Y/N #pk / sexual activity Y/N / etoh, other substances Y/N / occupation:
FAM HX	ca / HTN / MI / CAD / stroke / hyperlipidemia / DM2 / Alzheimer's / depression / osteoporosis / other:

GENERAL	well appearing / well nourished / a&o x 3 / normal mood / normal affect
NEURO	intact / abnormal **DTR:** 1 2 3 4 5 location:
SKIN + NAILS	turgor / rash / bruising / lesions // texture, distribution of hair // nails: abnormal color / nail deformity
HEAD	normocephalic / atraumatic / visible mass / palpable mass / depression / scarring
EYES	acuity intact / conjunctiva clear / EOM intact / PERRLA / fundi: normal discs and vessels / icterus / exudate / hemorrhage
EARS	EACs clear / TM translucent, mobile / landmarks abnormal / hearing diminished
NOSE	lesions / mucosal inflammation / septum, turbinates abnormal / sinus tenderness
MOUTH	mucous membranes dry / lesions / poor dentition / caries / gingival inflammation
PHARYNX	mucosa inflammation / tonsillar hypertrophy / tonsillar exudate
NECK	supple / ROM WNL / lesion / bruit / adenopathy / thyroid enlarged, tender / mass
CARDIAC	regular rate, rhythm / S1, S2 / murmur / gallop / click / rub / PMI displacement
RESP	clear to auscultation in all fields / wheezes (insp) (exp) / rales / crackles
ABDOMEN	BSx4 / tender / organomegaly / mass / hernia
RECTAL	abnormal tone / hemorrhoids (int/ext) / palpable mass
BACK	abnormal curvature / tenderness / CVAT / Δ ROM
EXTREMITIES	amputation / deformity / edema / varicosities / + pulses
MSK	abnormal gait / asymmetry / crepitation / defect / tenderness / mass / effusion / Δ ROM / instability / atrophy / abnormal strength, tone in head, neck, spine, ribs, pelvis, UE, LE / pathologic reflexes
PSYCH	A&O x3 / +recent/remote memory / insight / affect
BREAST	nipple abnormality / mass / tenderness / axillary, clavicular adenopathy
GYN/GU	lesions / d/c / uterus, adnexa tenderness / CMT // circumcised / penile lesions / urethra normal location, no d/c / testes normal / + cremasteric reflex
FEET	+ pulses / monofilament + / nails abnormal / dry, broken skin / callus

LABS	CBC / CMP / lipids / TSH / microalbumin / A1C / UA, culture / PSA / iron studies / other:

DIAGNOSTICS	XR / MRI / CT / US / cardiac / other
REFERRALS	**F/U** ___ wk ___ mo

| Patient ID#: | Date of visit: |
| Reason for visit: | Age: Gender: |

BP:	HT:
HR:	WT:
T:	BMI:
O2%:	PAIN:

NOTES . . . .

CONST	Δ appetite, energy, weight / fever / chills / sweats / fatigue
HEAD	trauma / mass / tenderness / rash / lesions
EYES	visionΔ / itch / d/c / tears / dry / cataracts / glaucoma / glasses, contacts
ENT	hearing Δ / pain / d/c / vertigo / ? infection // epistaxis / congestion // bleeding, swelling gums / pain / sore throat / voice Δ // neck pain / lumps / swelling / difficulty swallowing
CARDIAC	pain / pressure / dizzy / N / orthopnea / edema / palp / weak w exertion / hx murmurs / hx MI / HTN / HF / numb / tingle / cold extrem / slow wound healing
RESP	wheeze / SOB / cough / asthma / bronch / COPD
GI	abd pain / Δ in bowels / constipation / diarrhea / N V / hepatitis / gallstones / dysphagia / reflux / hemorrhoids / black, bloody stools
GU	burn / pain / nocturia / polyuria / hematuria / incontinence / infection / kid. stones
GENITAL	DC / sores / pain / masses / last pap _____ / sexually active Y N / dyspareunia / LMP _____ / contraception
MSK	redness / swelling / warmth / pain / +/- ROM / arthritis / musc cramps / fracture / sprains / joint replacement / stiffness: AM PM
SKIN	rash / pruritis / jaundice / bruising / hx skin ca / mole Δ / Δ in hair, nails / lesions / slow wound healing
BREASTS	lump / pain / dc / last mammo _____ / self exams YN
NEURO	HA / seizure / vertigo / memory Δ / gait Δ / speech / coord
PSYCH	depression / anxiety / Δ in sleep pattern / substance, ETOH abuse / suicidal ideation / homicidal ideation
ENDO	polydipsia, polyuria / heat, cold intolerance / Δ hair/nails/energy
HEM/LYMPH	anemia / bruising / hx transfusions / blood disorder / lymphadenopathy / axillary, groin tenderness
ALLX/IMMUN	season allx / food allx / med allx / immune disorder:

SOCIAL HX	# in household _____ / lives with SP/BF/GF/SO / children __ / tobacco Y/N #pk / sexual activity Y/N / etoh, other substances Y/N / occupation:
FAM HX	ca / HTN / MI / CAD / stroke / hyperlipidemia / DM2 / Alzheimer's / depression / osteoporosis / other:

GENERAL	well appearing / well nourished / a&o x 3 / normal mood / normal affect
NEURO	intact / abnormal **DTR:** 1 2 3 4 5 location:
SKIN + NAILS	turgor / rash / bruising / lesions // texture, distribution of hair // nails: abnormal color / nail deformity
HEAD	normocephalic / atraumatic / visible mass / palpable mass / depression / scarring
EYES	acuity intact / conjunctiva clear / EOM intact / PERRLA / fundi: normal discs and vessels / icterus / exudate / hemorrhage
EARS	EACs clear / TM translucent, mobile / landmarks abnormal / hearing diminished
NOSE	lesions / mucosal inflammation / septum, turbinates abnormal / sinus tenderness
MOUTH	mucous membranes dry / lesions / poor dentition / caries / gingival inflammation
PHARYNX	mucosa inflammation / tonsillar hypertrophy / tonsillar exudate
NECK	supple / ROM WNL / lesion / bruit / adenopathy / thyroid enlarged, tender / mass
CARDIAC	regular rate, rhythm / S1, S2 / murmur / gallop / click / rub / PMI displacement
RESP	clear to auscultation in all fields / wheezes (insp) (exp) / rales / crackles
ABDOMEN	BSx4 / tender / organomegaly / mass / hernia
RECTAL	abnormal tone / hemorrhoids (int/ext) / palpable mass
BACK	abnormal curvature / tenderness / CVAT / Δ ROM
EXTREMITIES	amputation / deformity / edema / varicosities / + pulses
MSK	abnormal gait / asymmetry / crepitation / defect / tenderness / mass / effusion / Δ ROM / instability / atrophy / abnormal strength, tone in head, neck, spine, ribs, pelvis, UE, LE / pathologic reflexes
PSYCH	A&O x3 / +recent/remote memory / insight / affect
BREAST	nipple abnormality / mass / tenderness / axillary, clavicular adenopathy
GYN/GU	lesions / d/c / uterus, adnexa tenderness / CMT // circumcised / penile lesions / urethra normal location, no d/c / testes normal / + cremasteric reflex
FEET	+ pulses / monofilament + / nails abnormal / dry, broken skin / callus

LABS	CBC / CMP / lipids / TSH / microalbumin / A1C / UA, culture / PSA / iron studies / other:
DIAGNOSTICS	XR / MRI / CT / US / cardiac / other
REFERRALS	**F/U** ___ wk ___ mo

<table>
<tr><td>

Patient ID#:	Date of visit:
Reason for visit:	Age: Gender:

</td><td>

BP: HT:
HR: WT:
T: BMI:
O2%:   PAIN:

NOTES . . . .

</td></tr>
</table>

CONST Δ appetite, energy, weight / fever / chills / sweats / fatigue

HEAD trauma / mass / tenderness / rash / lesions

EYES visionΔ / itch / d/c / tears / dry / cataracts / glaucoma / glasses, contacts

ENT hearing Δ / pain / d/c / vertigo / ? infection // epistaxis / congestion // bleeding, swelling gums / pain / sore throat / voice Δ // neck pain / lumps / swelling / difficulty swallowing

CARDIAC pain / pressure / dizzy / N / orthopnea / edema / palp / weak w exertion / hx murmurs / hx MI / HTN / HF / numb / tingle / cold extrem / slow wound healing

RESP wheeze / SOB / cough / asthma / bronch / COPD

GI abd pain / Δ in bowels / constipation / diarrhea / N V / hepatitis / gallstones / dysphagia / reflux / hemorrhoids / black, bloody stools

GU burn / pain / nocturia / polyuria / hematuria / incontinence / infection / kid. stones

GENITAL DC / sores / pain / masses / last pap _______ / sexually active Y N / dyspareunia / LMP _________ / contraception

MSK redness / swelling / warmth / pain / +/- ROM / arthritis / musc cramps / fracture / sprains / joint replacement / stiffness: AM PM

SKIN rash / pruritis / jaundice / bruising / hx skin ca / mole Δ / Δ in hair, nails / lesions / slow wound healing

BREASTS lump / pain / dc / last mammo ______ / self exams YN

NEURO HA / seizure / vertigo / memory Δ / gait Δ / speech / coord

PSYCH depression / anxiety / Δ in sleep pattern / substance, ETOH abuse / suicidal ideation / homicidal ideation

ENDO polydipsia, polyuria / heat, cold intolerance / Δ hair/nails/energy

HEM/LYMPH anemia / bruising / hx transfusions / blood disorder / lymphadenopathy / axillary, groin tenderness

ALLX/IMMUN season allx / food allx / med allx / immune disorder:

SOCIAL HX # in household ______ / lives with SP/BF/GF/SO / children __ / tobacco Y/N #pk / sexual activity Y/N / etoh, other substances Y/N / occupation:

FAM HX ca / HTN / MI / CAD / stroke / hyperlipidemia / DM2 / Alzheimer's / depression / osteoporosis / other:

GENERAL well appearing / well nourished / a&o x 3 / normal mood / normal affect

NEURO intact / abnormal   **DTR:** 1 2 3 4 5 location:

SKIN + NAILS turgor / rash / bruising / lesions // texture, distribution of hair // nails: abnormal color / nail deformity

HEAD normocephalic / atraumatic / visible mass / palpable mass / depression / scarring

EYES acuity intact / conjunctiva clear / EOM intact / PERRLA / fundi: normal discs and vessels / icterus / exudate / hemorrhage

EARS EACs clear / TM translucent, mobile / landmarks abnormal / hearing diminished

NOSE lesions / mucosal inflammation / septum, turbinates abnormal / sinus tenderness

MOUTH mucous membranes dry / lesions / poor dentition / caries / gingival inflammation

PHARYNX mucosa inflammation / tonsillar hypertrophy / tonsillar exudate

NECK supple / ROM WNL / lesion / bruit / adenopathy / thyroid enlarged, tender / mass

CARDIAC regular rate, rhythm / S1, S2 / murmur / gallop / click / rub / PMI displacement

RESP clear to auscultation in all fields / wheezes (insp) (exp) / rales / crackles

ABDOMEN BSx4 / tender / organomegaly / mass / hernia

RECTAL abnormal tone / hemorrhoids (int/ext) / palpable mass

BACK abnormal curvature / tenderness / CVAT / Δ ROM

EXTREMITIES amputation / deformity / edema / varicosities / + pulses

MSK abnormal gait / asymmetry / crepitation / defect / tenderness / mass / effusion / Δ ROM / instability / atrophy / abnormal strength, tone in head, neck, spine, ribs, pelvis, UE, LE / pathologic reflexes

PSYCH A&O x3 / +recent/remote memory / insight / affect

BREAST nipple abnormality / mass / tenderness / axillary, clavicular adenopathy

GYN/GU lesions / d/c / uterus, adnexa tenderness / CMT // circumcised / penile lesions / urethra normal location, no d/c / testes normal / + cremasteric reflex

FEET + pulses / monofilament + / nails abnormal / dry, broken skin / callus

---

LABS CBC / CMP / lipids / TSH / microalbumin / A1C / UA, culture / PSA / iron studies / other:

DIAGNOSTICS XR / MRI / CT / US / cardiac / other

REFERRALS   **F/U** ___ wk ___ mo

<table>
<tr><td>

Patient ID#:	Date of visit:
Reason for visit:	Age: Gender:

</td><td>

BP:	HT:
HR:	WT:
T:	BMI:
O2%:	PAIN:

NOTES . . . .

</td></tr>
</table>

CONST — Δ appetite, energy, weight / fever / chills / sweats / fatigue
HEAD — trauma / mass / tenderness / rash / lesions
EYES — visionΔ / itch / d/c / tears / dry / cataracts / glaucoma / glasses, contacts
ENT — hearing Δ / pain / d/c / vertigo / ? infection // epistaxis / congestion // bleeding, swelling gums / pain / sore throat / voice Δ // neck pain / lumps / swelling / difficulty swallowing

CARDIAC — pain / pressure / dizzy / N / orthopnea / edema / palp / weak w exertion / hx murmurs / hx MI / HTN / HF / numb / tingle / cold extrem / slow wound healing

RESP — wheeze / SOB / cough / asthma / bronch / COPD
GI — abd pain / Δ in bowels / constipation / diarrhea / N V / hepatitis / gallstones / dysphagia / reflux / hemorrhoids / black, bloody stools

GU — burn / pain / nocturia / polyuria / hematuria / incontinence / infection / kid. stones
GENITAL — DC / sores / pain / masses / last pap ______ / sexually active Y N / dyspareunia / LMP ______ / contraception

MSK — redness / swelling / warmth / pain / +/- ROM / arthritis / musc cramps / fracture / sprains / joint replacement / stiffness: AM PM

SKIN — rash / pruritis / jaundice / bruising / hx skin ca / mole Δ / Δ in hair, nails / lesions / slow wound healing

BREASTS — lump / pain / dc / last mammo ______ / self exams YN
NEURO — HA / seizure / vertigo / memory Δ / gait Δ / speech / coord
PSYCH — depression / anxiety / Δ in sleep pattern / substance, ETOH abuse / suicidal ideation / homicidal ideation

ENDO — polydipsia, polyuria / heat, cold intolerance / Δ hair/nails/energy
HEM/LYMPH — anemia / bruising / hx transfusions / blood disorder / lymphadenopathy / axillary, groin tenderness

ALLX/IMMUN — season allx / food allx / med allx / immune disorder:

SOCIAL HX — # in household ______ / lives with SP/BF/GF/SO / children __ / tobacco Y/N #pk / sexual activity Y/N / etoh, other substances Y/N / occupation:

FAM HX — ca / HTN / MI / CAD / stroke / hyperlipidemia / DM2 / Alzheimer's / depression / osteoporosis / other:

GENERAL — well appearing / well nourished / a&o x 3 / normal mood / normal affect
NEURO — intact / abnormal   **DTR:** 1 2 3 4 5 location:
SKIN + NAILS — turgor / rash / bruising / lesions // texture, distribution of hair // nails: abnormal color / nail deformity

HEAD — normocephalic / atraumatic / visible mass / palpable mass / depression / scarring
EYES — acuity intact / conjunctiva clear / EOM intact / PERRLA / fundi: normal discs and vessels / icterus / exudate / hemorrhage

EARS — EACs clear / TM translucent, mobile / landmarks abnormal / hearing diminished
NOSE — lesions / mucosal inflammation / septum, turbinates abnormal / sinus tenderness
MOUTH — mucous membranes dry / lesions / poor dentition / caries / gingival inflammation
PHARYNX — mucosa inflammation / tonsillar hypertrophy / tonsillar exudate
NECK — supple / ROM WNL / lesion / bruit / adenopathy / thyroid enlarged, tender / mass
CARDIAC — regular rate, rhythm / S1, S2 / murmur / gallop / click / rub / PMI displacement
RESP — clear to auscultation in all fields / wheezes (insp) (exp) / rales / crackles
ABDOMEN — BSx4 / tender / organomegaly / mass / hernia
RECTAL — abnormal tone / hemorrhoids (int/ext) / palpable mass
BACK — abnormal curvature / tenderness / CVAT / Δ ROM
EXTREMITIES — amputation / deformity / edema / varicosities / + pulses
MSK — abnormal gait / asymmetry / crepitation / defect / tenderness / mass / effusion / Δ ROM / instability / atrophy / abnormal strength, tone in head, neck, spine, ribs, pelvis, UE, LE / pathologic reflexes

PSYCH — A&O x3 / +recent/remote memory / insight / affect
BREAST — nipple abnormality / mass / tenderness / axillary, clavicular adenopathy
GYN/GU — lesions / d/c / uterus, adnexa tenderness / CMT // circumcised / penile lesions / urethra normal location, no d/c / testes normal / + cremasteric reflex

FEET — + pulses / monofilament + / nails abnormal / dry, broken skin / callus

---

LABS — CBC / CMP / lipids / TSH / microalbumin / A1C / UA, culture / PSA / iron studies / other:

DIAGNOSTICS — XR / MRI / CT / US / cardiac / other
REFERRALS —   **F/U** ___ wk ___ mo

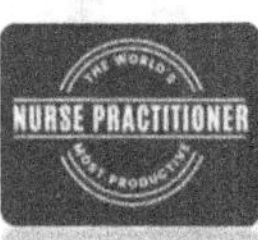

<table>
<tr><td>

Patient ID#:   **Date of visit:**
Reason for visit: **Age:**   **Gender:**

</td><td>

BP: HT:
HR: WT:
T: BMI:
O2%:   PAIN:

NOTES . . . .

</td></tr>
</table>

CONST	Δ appetite, energy, weight / fever / chills / sweats / fatigue
HEAD	trauma / mass / tenderness / rash / lesions
EYES	visionΔ / itch / d/c / tears / dry / cataracts / glaucoma / glasses, contacts
ENT	hearing Δ / pain / d/c / vertigo / ? infection // epistaxis / congestion // bleeding, swelling gums / pain / sore throat / voice Δ // neck pain / lumps / swelling / difficulty swallowing
CARDIAC	pain / pressure / dizzy / N / orthopnea / edema / palp / weak w exertion / hx murmurs / hx MI / HTN / HF / numb / tingle / cold extrem / slow wound healing
RESP	wheeze / SOB / cough / asthma / bronch / COPD
GI	abd pain / Δ in bowels / constipation / diarrhea / N V / hepatitis / gallstones / dysphagia / reflux / hemorrhoids / black, bloody stools
GU	burn / pain / nocturia / polyuria / hematuria / incontinence / infection / kid. stones
GENITAL	DC / sores / pain / masses / last pap ______ / sexually active Y N / dyspareunia / LMP ______ / contraception
MSK	redness / swelling / warmth / pain / +/- ROM / arthritis / musc cramps / fracture / sprains / joint replacement / stiffness: AM PM
SKIN	rash / pruritis / jaundice / bruising / hx skin ca / mole Δ / Δ in hair, nails / lesions / slow wound healing
BREASTS	lump / pain / dc / last mammo ______ / self exams YN
NEURO	HA / seizure / vertigo / memory Δ / gait Δ / speech / coord
PSYCH	depression / anxiety / Δ in sleep pattern / substance, ETOH abuse / suicidal ideation / homicidal ideation
ENDO	polydipsia, polyuria / heat, cold intolerance / Δ hair/nails/energy
HEM/LYMPH	anemia / bruising / hx transfusions / blood disorder / lymphadenopathy / axillary, groin tenderness
ALLX/IMMUN	season allx / food allx / med allx / immune disorder:

SOCIAL HX	# in household ______ / lives with SP/BF/GF/SO / children __ / tobacco Y/N #pk / sexual activity Y/N / etoh, other substances Y/N / occupation:
FAM HX	ca / HTN / MI / CAD / stroke / hyperlipidemia / DM2 / Alzheimer's / depression / osteoporosis / other:

GENERAL	well appearing / well nourished / a&o x 3 / normal mood / normal affect
NEURO	intact / abnormal **DTR:** 1 2 3 4 5 location:
SKIN + NAILS	turgor / rash / bruising / lesions // texture, distribution of hair // nails: abnormal color / nail deformity
HEAD	normocephalic / atraumatic / visible mass / palpable mass / depression / scarring
EYES	acuity intact / conjunctiva clear / EOM intact / PERRLA / fundi: normal discs and vessels / icterus / exudate / hemorrhage
EARS	EACs clear / TM translucent, mobile / landmarks abnormal / hearing diminished
NOSE	lesions / mucosal inflammation / septum, turbinates abnormal / sinus tenderness
MOUTH	mucous membranes dry / lesions / poor dentition / caries / gingival inflammation
PHARYNX	mucosa inflammation / tonsillar hypertrophy / tonsillar exudate
NECK	supple / ROM WNL / lesion / bruit / adenopathy / thyroid enlarged, tender / mass
CARDIAC	regular rate, rhythm / S1, S2 / murmur / gallop / click / rub / PMI displacement
RESP	clear to auscultation in all fields / wheezes (insp) (exp) / rales / crackles
ABDOMEN	BSx4 / tender / organomegaly / mass / hernia
RECTAL	abnormal tone / hemorrhoids (int/ext) / palpable mass
BACK	abnormal curvature / tenderness / CVAT / Δ ROM
EXTREMITIES	amputation / deformity / edema / varicosities / + pulses
MSK	abnormal gait / asymmetry / crepitation / defect / tenderness / mass / effusion / Δ ROM / instability / atrophy / abnormal strength, tone in head, neck, spine, ribs, pelvis, UE, LE / pathologic reflexes
PSYCH	A&O x3 / +recent/remote memory / insight / affect
BREAST	nipple abnormality / mass / tenderness / axillary, clavicular adenopathy
GYN/GU	lesions / d/c / uterus, adnexa tenderness / CMT // circumcised / penile lesions / urethra normal location, no d/c / testes normal / + cremasteric reflex
FEET	+ pulses / monofilament + / nails abnormal / dry, broken skin / callus

LABS	CBC / CMP / lipids / TSH / microalbumin / A1C / UA, culture / PSA / iron studies / other:

DIAGNOSTICS	XR / MRI / CT / US / cardiac / other
REFERRALS	**F/U** ___ wk ___ mo

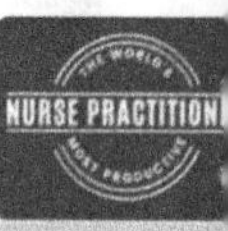

BP:	HT:
HR:	WT:
T:	BMI:
O2%:	PAIN:

Patient ID#:		**Date of visit:**	
Reason for visit:		**Age:**	**Gender:**

NOTES . . . .

CONST Δ appetite, energy, weight / fever / chills / sweats / fatigue
HEAD trauma / mass / tenderness / rash / lesions
EYES visionΔ / itch / d/c / tears / dry / cataracts / glaucoma / glasses, contacts
ENT hearing Δ / pain / d/c / vertigo / ? infection // epistaxis / congestion // bleeding, swelling gums / pain / sore throat / voice Δ // neck pain / lumps / swelling / difficulty swallowing

CARDIAC pain / pressure / dizzy / N / orthopnea / edema / palp / weak w exertion / hx murmurs / hx MI / HTN / HF / numb / tingle / cold extrem / slow wound healing

RESP wheeze / SOB / cough / asthma / bronch / COPD
GI abd pain / Δ in bowels / constipation / diarrhea / N V / hepatitis / gallstones / dysphagia / reflux / hemorrhoids / black, bloody stools

GU burn / pain / nocturia / polyuria / hematuria / incontinence / infection / kid. stones
GENITAL DC / sores / pain / masses / last pap _____ / sexually active Y N / dyspareunia / LMP _______ / contraception

MSK redness / swelling / warmth / pain / +/- ROM / arthritis / musc cramps / fracture / sprains / joint replacement / stiffness: AM PM
SKIN rash / pruritis / jaundice / bruising / hx skin ca / mole Δ / Δ in hair, nails / lesions / slow wound healing

BREASTS lump / pain / dc / last mammo _______ / self exams YN
NEURO HA / seizure / vertigo / memory Δ / gait Δ / speech / coord
PSYCH depression / anxiety / Δ in sleep pattern / substance, ETOH abuse / suicidal ideation / homicidal ideation

ENDO polydipsia, polyuria / heat, cold intolerance / Δ hair/nails/energy
HEM/LYMPH anemia / bruising / hx transfusions / blood disorder / lymphadenopathy / axillary, groin tenderness

ALLX/IMMUN season allx / food allx / med allx / immune disorder:

SOCIAL HX # in household _______ / lives with SP/BF/GF/SO / children __ / tobacco Y/N #pk / sexual activity Y/N / etoh, other substances Y/N / occupation:
FAM HX ca / HTN / MI / CAD / stroke / hyperlipidemia / DM2 / Alzheimer's / depression / osteoporosis / other:

GENERAL well appearing / well nourished / a&o x 3 / normal mood / normal affect
NEURO intact / abnormal **DTR:** 1 2 3 4 5 location:
SKIN + NAILS turgor / rash / bruising / lesions // texture, distribution of hair // nails: abnormal color / nail deformity

HEAD normocephalic / atraumatic / visible mass / palpable mass / depression / scarring
EYES acuity intact / conjunctiva clear / EOM intact / PERRLA / fundi: normal discs and vessels / icterus / exudate / hemorrhage

EARS EACs clear / TM translucent, mobile / landmarks abnormal / hearing diminished
NOSE lesions / mucosal inflammation / septum, turbinates abnormal / sinus tenderness
MOUTH mucous membranes dry / lesions / poor dentition / caries / gingival inflammation
PHARYNX mucosa inflammation / tonsillar hypertrophy / tonsillar exudate
NECK supple / ROM WNL / lesion / bruit / adenopathy / thyroid enlarged, tender / mass
CARDIAC regular rate, rhythm / S1, S2 / murmur / gallop / click / rub / PMI displacement
RESP clear to auscultation in all fields / wheezes (insp) (exp) / rales / crackles
ABDOMEN BSx4 / tender / organomegaly / mass / hernia
RECTAL abnormal tone / hemorrhoids (int/ext) / palpable mass
BACK abnormal curvature / tenderness / CVAT / Δ ROM
EXTREMITIES amputation / deformity / edema / varicosities / + pulses
MSK abnormal gait / asymmetry / crepitation / defect / tenderness / mass / effusion / Δ ROM / instability / atrophy / abnormal strength, tone in head, neck, spine, ribs, pelvis, UE, LE / pathologic reflexes

PSYCH A&O x3 / +recent/remote memory / insight / affect
BREAST nipple abnormality / mass / tenderness / axillary, clavicular adenopathy
GYN/GU lesions / d/c / uterus, adnexa tenderness / CMT // circumcised / penile lesions / urethra normal location, no d/c / testes normal / + cremasteric reflex
FEET + pulses / monofilament + / nails abnormal / dry, broken skin / callus

---

LABS CBC / CMP / lipids / TSH / microalbumin / A1C / UA, culture / PSA / iron studies / other:

DIAGNOSTICS XR / MRI / CT / US / cardiac / other
REFERRALS **F/U** ___ wk ___ mo

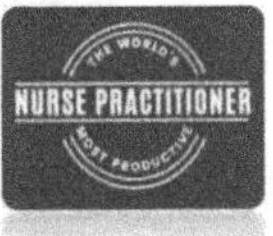

<table>
<tr><td colspan="2">Patient ID#:
Reason for visit:</td><td>Date of visit:
Age: Gender:</td></tr>
</table>

BP: HT:
HR: WT:
T: BMI:
O2%:   PAIN:

NOTES . . . .

CONST	Δ appetite, energy, weight / fever / chills / sweats / fatigue
HEAD	trauma / mass / tenderness / rash / lesions
EYES	visionΔ / itch / d/c / tears / dry / cataracts / glaucoma / glasses, contacts
ENT	hearing Δ / pain / d/c / vertigo / ? infection // epistaxis / congestion // bleeding, swelling gums / pain / sore throat / voice Δ // neck pain / lumps / swelling / difficulty swallowing
CARDIAC	pain / pressure / dizzy / N / orthopnea / edema / palp / weak w exertion / hx murmurs / hx MI / HTN / HF / numb / tingle / cold extrem / slow wound healing
RESP	wheeze / SOB / cough / asthma / bronch / COPD
GI	abd pain / Δ in bowels / constipation / diarrhea / N V / hepatitis / gallstones / dysphagia / reflux / hemorrhoids / black, bloody stools
GU	burn / pain / nocturia / polyuria / hematuria / incontinence / infection / kid. stones
GENITAL	DC / sores / pain / masses / last pap _____ / sexually active Y N / dyspareunia / LMP _____ / contraception
MSK	redness / swelling / warmth / pain / +/- ROM / arthritis / musc cramps / fracture / sprains / joint replacement / stiffness: AM PM
SKIN	rash / pruritis / jaundice / bruising / hx skin ca / mole Δ / Δ in hair, nails / lesions / slow wound healing
BREASTS	lump / pain / dc / last mammo _____ / self exams YN
NEURO	HA / seizure / vertigo / memory Δ / gait Δ / speech / coord
PSYCH	depression / anxiety / Δ in sleep pattern / substance, ETOH abuse / suicidal ideation / homicidal ideation
ENDO	polydipsia, polyuria / heat, cold intolerance / Δ hair/nails/energy
HEM/LYMPH	anemia / bruising / hx transfusions / blood disorder / lymphadenopathy / axillary, groin tenderness
ALLX/IMMUN	season allx / food allx / med allx / immune disorder:

SOCIAL HX	# in household _____ / lives with SP/BF/GF/SO / children __ / tobacco Y/N #pk / sexual activity Y/N / etoh, other substances Y/N / occupation:
FAM HX	ca / HTN / MI / CAD / stroke / hyperlipidemia / DM2 / Alzheimer's / depression / osteoporosis / other:

GENERAL	well appearing / well nourished / a&o x 3 / normal mood / normal affect
NEURO	intact / abnormal **DTR:** 1 2 3 4 5 location:
SKIN + NAILS	turgor / rash / bruising / lesions // texture, distribution of hair // nails: abnormal color / nail deformity
HEAD	normocephalic / atraumatic / visible mass / palpable mass / depression / scarring
EYES	acuity intact / conjunctiva clear / EOM intact / PERRLA / fundi: normal discs and vessels / icterus / exudate / hemorrhage
EARS	EACs clear / TM translucent, mobile / landmarks abnormal / hearing diminished
NOSE	lesions / mucosal inflammation / septum, turbinates abnormal / sinus tenderness
MOUTH	mucous membranes dry / lesions / poor dentition / caries / gingival inflammation
PHARYNX	mucosa inflammation / tonsillar hypertrophy / tonsillar exudate
NECK	supple / ROM WNL / lesion / bruit / adenopathy / thyroid enlarged, tender / mass
CARDIAC	regular rate, rhythm / S1, S2 / murmur / gallop / click / rub / PMI displacement
RESP	clear to auscultation in all fields / wheezes (insp) (exp) / rales / crackles
ABDOMEN	BSx4 / tender / organomegaly / mass / hernia
RECTAL	abnormal tone / hemorrhoids (int/ext) / palpable mass
BACK	abnormal curvature / tenderness / CVAT / Δ ROM
EXTREMITIES	amputation / deformity / edema / varicosities / + pulses
MSK	abnormal gait / asymmetry / crepitation / defect / tenderness / mass / effusion / Δ ROM / instability / atrophy / abnormal strength, tone in head, neck, spine, ribs, pelvis, UE, LE / pathologic reflexes
PSYCH	A&O x3 / +recent/remote memory / insight / affect
BREAST	nipple abnormality / mass / tenderness / axillary, clavicular adenopathy
GYN/GU	lesions / d/c / uterus, adnexa tenderness / CMT // circumcised / penile lesions / urethra normal location, no d/c / testes normal / + cremasteric reflex
FEET	+ pulses / monofilament + / nails abnormal / dry, broken skin / callus

LABS	CBC / CMP / lipids / TSH / microalbumin / A1C / UA, culture / PSA / iron studies / other:

DIAGNOSTICS	XR / MRI / CT / US / cardiac / other
REFERRALS	**F/U** ___ wk ___ mo

| Patient ID#: | Date of visit: |
| Reason for visit: | Age: Gender: |

BP:	HT:
HR:	WT:
T:	BMI:
O2%:	PAIN:

NOTES . . . .

CONST	Δ appetite, energy, weight / fever / chills / sweats / fatigue
HEAD	trauma / mass / tenderness / rash / lesions
EYES	visionΔ / itch / d/c / tears / dry / cataracts / glaucoma / glasses, contacts
ENT	hearing Δ / pain / d/c / vertigo / ? infection // epistaxis / congestion // bleeding, swelling gums / pain / sore throat / voice Δ // neck pain / lumps / swelling / difficulty swallowing
CARDIAC	pain / pressure / dizzy / N / orthopnea / edema / palp / weak w exertion / hx murmurs / hx MI / HTN / HF / numb / tingle / cold extrem / slow wound healing
RESP	wheeze / SOB / cough / asthma / bronch / COPD
GI	abd pain / Δ in bowels / constipation / diarrhea / N V / hepatitis / gallstones / dysphagia / reflux / hemorrhoids / black, bloody stools
GU	burn / pain / nocturia / polyuria / hematuria / incontinence / infection / kid. stones
GENITAL	DC / sores / pain / masses / last pap ______ / sexually active Y N / dyspareunia / LMP ______ / contraception
MSK	redness / swelling / warmth / pain / +/- ROM / arthritis / musc cramps / fracture / sprains / joint replacement / stiffness: AM PM
SKIN	rash / pruritis / jaundice / bruising / hx skin ca / mole Δ / Δ in hair, nails / lesions / slow wound healing
BREASTS	lump / pain / dc / last mammo ______ / self exams YN
NEURO	HA / seizure / vertigo / memory Δ / gait Δ / speech / coord
PSYCH	depression / anxiety / Δ in sleep pattern / substance, ETOH abuse / suicidal ideation / homicidal ideation
ENDO	polydipsia, polyuria / heat, cold intolerance / Δ hair/nails/energy
HEM/LYMPH	anemia / bruising / hx transfusions / blood disorder / lymphadenopathy / axillary, groin tenderness
ALLX/IMMUN	season allx / food allx / med allx / immune disorder:

SOCIAL HX	# in household ______ / lives with SP/BF/GF/SO / children __ / tobacco Y/N #pk / sexual activity Y/N / etoh, other substances Y/N / occupation:
FAM HX	ca / HTN / MI / CAD / stroke / hyperlipidemia / DM2 / Alzheimer's / depression / osteoporosis / other:

GENERAL	well appearing / well nourished / a&o x 3 / normal mood / normal affect
NEURO	intact / abnormal **DTR:** 1 2 3 4 5 location:
SKIN + NAILS	turgor / rash / bruising / lesions // texture, distribution of hair // nails: abnormal color / nail deformity
HEAD	normocephalic / atraumatic / visible mass / palpable mass / depression / scarring
EYES	acuity intact / conjunctiva clear / EOM intact / PERRLA / fundi: normal discs and vessels / icterus / exudate / hemorrhage
EARS	EACs clear / TM translucent, mobile / landmarks abnormal / hearing diminished
NOSE	lesions / mucosal inflammation / septum, turbinates abnormal / sinus tenderness
MOUTH	mucous membranes dry / lesions / poor dentition / caries / gingival inflammation
PHARYNX	mucosa inflammation / tonsillar hypertrophy / tonsillar exudate
NECK	supple / ROM WNL / lesion / bruit / adenopathy / thyroid enlarged, tender / mass
CARDIAC	regular rate, rhythm / S1, S2 / murmur / gallop / click / rub / PMI displacement
RESP	clear to auscultation in all fields / wheezes (insp) (exp) / rales / crackles
ABDOMEN	BSx4 / tender / organomegaly / mass / hernia
RECTAL	abnormal tone / hemorrhoids (int/ext) / palpable mass
BACK	abnormal curvature / tenderness / CVAT / Δ ROM
EXTREMITIES	amputation / deformity / edema / varicosities / + pulses
MSK	abnormal gait / asymmetry / crepitation / defect / tenderness / mass / effusion / Δ ROM / instability / atrophy / abnormal strength, tone in head, neck, spine, ribs, pelvis, UE, LE / pathologic reflexes
PSYCH	A&O x3 / +recent/remote memory / insight / affect
BREAST	nipple abnormality / mass / tenderness / axillary, clavicular adenopathy
GYN/GU	lesions / d/c / uterus, adnexa tenderness / CMT // circumcised / penile lesions / urethra normal location, no d/c / testes normal / + cremasteric reflex
FEET	+ pulses / monofilament + / nails abnormal / dry, broken skin / callus

LABS	CBC / CMP / lipids / TSH / microalbumin / A1C / UA, culture / PSA / iron studies / other:

DIAGNOSTICS	XR / MRI / CT / US / cardiac / other
REFERRALS	**F/U** ___ wk ___ mo

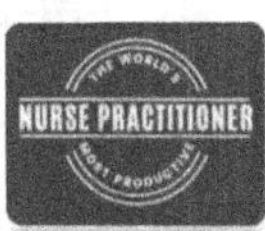

<table>
<tr><td>Patient ID#:</td><td>Date of visit:</td></tr>
<tr><td>Reason for visit:</td><td>Age: Gender:</td></tr>
</table>

BP: HT:
HR: WT:
T: BMI:
O2%:   PAIN:

NOTES . . . .

CONST	Δ appetite, energy, weight / fever / chills / sweats / fatigue
HEAD	trauma / mass / tenderness / rash / lesions
EYES	visionΔ / itch / d/c / tears / dry / cataracts / glaucoma / glasses, contacts
ENT	hearing Δ / pain / d/c / vertigo / ? infection // epistaxis / congestion // bleeding, swelling gums / pain / sore throat / voice Δ // neck pain / lumps / swelling / difficulty swallowing
CARDIAC	pain / pressure / dizzy / N / orthopnea / edema / palp / weak w exertion / hx murmurs / hx MI / HTN / HF / numb / tingle / cold extrem / slow wound healing
RESP	wheeze / SOB / cough / asthma / bronch / COPD
GI	abd pain / Δ in bowels / constipation / diarrhea / N V / hepatitis / gallstones / dysphagia / reflux / hemorrhoids / black, bloody stools
GU	burn / pain / nocturia / polyuria / hematuria / incontinence / infection / kid. stones
GENITAL	DC / sores / pain / masses / last pap _____ / sexually active Y N / dyspareunia / LMP _____ / contraception
MSK	redness / swelling / warmth / pain / +/- ROM / arthritis / musc cramps / fracture / sprains / joint replacement / stiffness: AM PM
SKIN	rash / pruritis / jaundice / bruising / hx skin ca / mole Δ / Δ in hair, nails / lesions / slow wound healing
BREASTS	lump / pain / dc / last mammo _____ / self exams YN
NEURO	HA / seizure / vertigo / memory Δ / gait Δ / speech / coord
PSYCH	depression / anxiety / Δ in sleep pattern / substance, ETOH abuse / suicidal ideation / homicidal ideation
ENDO	polydipsia, polyuria / heat, cold intolerance / Δ hair/nails/energy
HEM/LYMPH	anemia / bruising / hx transfusions / blood disorder / lymphadenopathy / axillary, groin tenderness
ALLX/IMMUN	season allx / food allx / med allx / immune disorder:

SOCIAL HX	# in household _____ / lives with SP/BF/GF/SO / children __ / tobacco Y/N #pk / sexual activity Y/N / etoh, other substances Y/N / occupation:
FAM HX	ca / HTN / MI / CAD / stroke / hyperlipidemia / DM2 / Alzheimer's / depression / osteoporosis / other:

GENERAL	well appearing / well nourished / a&o x 3 / normal mood / normal affect
NEURO	intact / abnormal **DTR:** 1 2 3 4 5 location:
SKIN + NAILS	turgor / rash / bruising / lesions // texture, distribution of hair // nails: abnormal color / nail deformity
HEAD	normocephalic / atraumatic / visible mass / palpable mass / depression / scarring
EYES	acuity intact / conjunctiva clear / EOM intact / PERRLA / fundi: normal discs and vessels / icterus / exudate / hemorrhage
EARS	EACs clear / TM translucent, mobile / landmarks abnormal / hearing diminished
NOSE	lesions / mucosal inflammation / septum, turbinates abnormal / sinus tenderness
MOUTH	mucous membranes dry / lesions / poor dentition / caries / gingival inflammation
PHARYNX	mucosa inflammation / tonsillar hypertrophy / tonsillar exudate
NECK	supple / ROM WNL / lesion / bruit / adenopathy / thyroid enlarged, tender / mass
CARDIAC	regular rate, rhythm / S1, S2 / murmur / gallop / click / rub / PMI displacement
RESP	clear to auscultation in all fields / wheezes (insp) (exp) / rales / crackles
ABDOMEN	BSx4 / tender / organomegaly / mass / hernia
RECTAL	abnormal tone / hemorrhoids (int/ext) / palpable mass
BACK	abnormal curvature / tenderness / CVAT / Δ ROM
EXTREMITIES	amputation / deformity / edema / varicosities / + pulses
MSK	abnormal gait / asymmetry / crepitation / defect / tenderness / mass / effusion / Δ ROM / instability / atrophy / abnormal strength, tone in head, neck, spine, ribs, pelvis, UE, LE / pathologic reflexes
PSYCH	A&O x3 / +recent/remote memory / insight / affect
BREAST	nipple abnormality / mass / tenderness / axillary, clavicular adenopathy
GYN/GU	lesions / d/c / uterus, adnexa tenderness / CMT // circumcised / penile lesions / urethra normal location, no d/c / testes normal / + cremasteric reflex
FEET	+ pulses / monofilament + / nails abnormal / dry, broken skin / callus

LABS	CBC / CMP / lipids / TSH / microalbumin / A1C / UA, culture / PSA / iron studies / other:

DIAGNOSTICS	XR / MRI / CT / US / cardiac / other
REFERRALS	**F/U** ___ wk ___ mo

<table>
<tr><td colspan="2">

Patient ID#:
Reason for visit:

</td><td>

Date of visit:
Age: Gender:

</td></tr>
</table>

BP:	**HT:**
HR:	**WT:**
T:	**BMI:**
O2%:	**PAIN:**

NOTES . . . .

CONST	Δ appetite, energy, weight / fever / chills / sweats / fatigue
HEAD	trauma / mass / tenderness / rash / lesions
EYES	visionΔ / itch / d/c / tears / dry / cataracts / glaucoma / glasses, contacts
ENT	hearing Δ / pain / d/c / vertigo / ? infection // epistaxis / congestion // bleeding, swelling gums / pain / sore throat / voice Δ // neck pain / lumps / swelling / difficulty swallowing
CARDIAC	pain / pressure / dizzy / N / orthopnea / edema / palp / weak w exertion / hx murmurs / hx MI / HTN / HF / numb / tingle / cold extrem / slow wound healing
RESP	wheeze / SOB / cough / asthma / bronch / COPD
GI	abd pain / Δ in bowels / constipation / diarrhea / N V / hepatitis / gallstones / dysphagia / reflux / hemorrhoids / black, bloody stools
GU	burn / pain / nocturia / polyuria / hematuria / incontinence / infection / kid. stones
GENITAL	DC / sores / pain / masses / last pap _____ / sexually active Y N / dyspareunia / LMP _____ / contraception
MSK	redness / swelling / warmth / pain / +/- ROM / arthritis / musc cramps / fracture / sprains / joint replacement / stiffness: AM PM
SKIN	rash / pruritis / jaundice / bruising / hx skin ca / mole Δ / Δ in hair, nails / lesions / slow wound healing
BREASTS	lump / pain / dc / last mammo _____ / self exams YN
NEURO	HA / seizure / vertigo / memory Δ / gait Δ / speech / coord
PSYCH	depression / anxiety / Δ in sleep pattern / substance, ETOH abuse / suicidal ideation / homicidal ideation
ENDO	polydipsia, polyuria / heat, cold intolerance / Δ hair/nails/energy
HEM/LYMPH	anemia / bruising / hx transfusions / blood disorder / lymphadenopathy / axillary, groin tenderness
ALLX/IMMUN	season allx / food allx / med allx / immune disorder:

SOCIAL HX	# in household _____ / lives with SP/BF/GF/SO / children __ / tobacco Y/N #pk / sexual activity Y/N / etoh, other substances Y/N / occupation:
FAM HX	ca / HTN / MI / CAD / stroke / hyperlipidemia / DM2 / Alzheimer's / depression / osteoporosis / other:

GENERAL	well appearing / well nourished / a&o x 3 / normal mood / normal affect
NEURO	intact / abnormal **DTR:** 1 2 3 4 5 location:
SKIN + NAILS	turgor / rash / bruising / lesions // texture, distribution of hair // nails: abnormal color / nail deformity
HEAD	normocephalic / atraumatic / visible mass / palpable mass / depression / scarring
EYES	acuity intact / conjunctiva clear / EOM intact / PERRLA / fundi: normal discs and vessels / icterus / exudate / hemorrhage
EARS	EACs clear / TM translucent, mobile / landmarks abnormal / hearing diminished
NOSE	lesions / mucosal inflammation / septum, turbinates abnormal / sinus tenderness
MOUTH	mucous membranes dry / lesions / poor dentition / caries / gingival inflammation
PHARYNX	mucosa inflammation / tonsillar hypertrophy / tonsillar exudate
NECK	supple / ROM WNL / lesion / bruit / adenopathy / thyroid enlarged, tender / mass
CARDIAC	regular rate, rhythm / S1, S2 / murmur / gallop / click / rub / PMI displacement
RESP	clear to auscultation in all fields / wheezes (insp) (exp) / rales / crackles
ABDOMEN	BSx4 / tender / organomegaly / mass / hernia
RECTAL	abnormal tone / hemorrhoids (int/ext) / palpable mass
BACK	abnormal curvature / tenderness / CVAT / Δ ROM
EXTREMITIES	amputation / deformity / edema / varicosities / + pulses
MSK	abnormal gait / asymmetry / crepitation / defect / tenderness / mass / effusion / Δ ROM / instability / atrophy / abnormal strength, tone in head, neck, spine, ribs, pelvis, UE, LE / pathologic reflexes
PSYCH	A&O x3 / +recent/remote memory / insight / affect
BREAST	nipple abnormality / mass / tenderness / axillary, clavicular adenopathy
GYN/GU	lesions / d/c / uterus, adnexa tenderness / CMT // circumcised / penile lesions / urethra normal location, no d/c / testes normal / + cremasteric reflex
FEET	+ pulses / monofilament + / nails abnormal / dry, broken skin / callus

LABS	CBC / CMP / lipids / TSH / microalbumin / A1C / UA, culture / PSA / iron studies / other:

DIAGNOSTICS	XR / MRI / CT / US / cardiac / other
REFERRALS	**F/U** ___ wk ___ mo

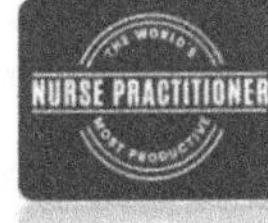

<table>
<tr><td colspan="2">

Patient ID#:

Reason for visit:
</td><td>

Date of visit:

Age: Gender:
</td></tr>
</table>

<table>
<tr><td>BP:</td><td>HT:</td></tr>
<tr><td>HR:</td><td>WT:</td></tr>
<tr><td>T:</td><td>BMI:</td></tr>
<tr><td>O2%:</td><td>PAIN:</td></tr>
</table>

NOTES . . . .

CONST — Δ appetite, energy, weight / fever / chills / sweats / fatigue

HEAD — trauma / mass / tenderness / rash / lesions

EYES — visionΔ / itch / d/c / tears / dry / cataracts / glaucoma / glasses, contacts

ENT — hearing Δ / pain / d/c / vertigo / ? infection // epistaxis / congestion // bleeding, swelling gums / pain / sore throat / voice Δ // neck pain / lumps / swelling / difficulty swallowing

CARDIAC — pain / pressure / dizzy / N / orthopnea / edema / palp / weak w exertion / hx murmurs / hx MI / HTN / HF / numb / tingle / cold extrem / slow wound healing

RESP — wheeze / SOB / cough / asthma / bronch / COPD

GI — abd pain / Δ in bowels / constipation / diarrhea / N V / hepatitis / gallstones / dysphagia / reflux / hemorrhoids / black, bloody stools

GU — burn / pain / nocturia / polyuria / hematuria / incontinence / infection / kid. stones

GENITAL — DC / sores / pain / masses / last pap ______ / sexually active Y N / dyspareunia / LMP ______ / contraception

MSK — redness / swelling / warmth / pain / +/- ROM / arthritis / musc cramps / fracture / sprains / joint replacement / stiffness: AM PM

SKIN — rash / pruritis / jaundice / bruising / hx skin ca / mole Δ / Δ in hair, nails / lesions / slow wound healing

BREASTS — lump / pain / dc / last mammo ______ / self exams YN

NEURO — HA / seizure / vertigo / memory Δ / gait Δ / speech / coord

PSYCH — depression / anxiety / Δ in sleep pattern / substance, ETOH abuse / suicidal ideation / homicidal ideation

ENDO — polydipsia, polyuria / heat, cold intolerance / Δ hair/nails/energy

HEM/LYMPH — anemia / bruising / hx transfusions / blood disorder / lymphadenopathy / axillary, groin tenderness

ALLX/IMMUN — season allx / food allx / med allx / immune disorder:

SOCIAL HX — # in household ______ / lives with SP/BF/GF/SO / children __ / tobacco Y/N #pk / sexual activity Y/N / etoh, other substances Y/N / occupation:

FAM HX — ca / HTN / MI / CAD / stroke / hyperlipidemia / DM2 / Alzheimer's / depression / osteoporosis / other:

GENERAL — well appearing / well nourished / a&o x 3 / normal mood / normal affect

NEURO — intact / abnormal   **DTR:** 1 2 3 4 5 location:

SKIN + NAILS — turgor / rash / bruising / lesions // texture, distribution of hair // nails: abnormal color / nail deformity

HEAD — normocephalic / atraumatic / visible mass / palpable mass / depression / scarring

EYES — acuity intact / conjunctiva clear / EOM intact / PERRLA / fundi: normal discs and vessels / icterus / exudate / hemorrhage

EARS — EACs clear / TM translucent, mobile / landmarks abnormal / hearing diminished

NOSE — lesions / mucosal inflammation / septum, turbinates abnormal / sinus tenderness

MOUTH — mucous membranes dry / lesions / poor dentition / caries / gingival inflammation

PHARYNX — mucosa inflammation / tonsillar hypertrophy / tonsillar exudate

NECK — supple / ROM WNL / lesion / bruit / adenopathy / thyroid enlarged, tender / mass

CARDIAC — regular rate, rhythm / S1, S2 / murmur / gallop / click / rub / PMI displacement

RESP — clear to auscultation in all fields / wheezes (insp) (exp) / rales / crackles

ABDOMEN — BSx4 / tender / organomegaly / mass / hernia

RECTAL — abnormal tone / hemorrhoids (int/ext) / palpable mass

BACK — abnormal curvature / tenderness / CVAT / Δ ROM

EXTREMITIES — amputation / deformity / edema / varicosities / + pulses

MSK — abnormal gait / asymmetry / crepitation / defect / tenderness / mass / effusion / Δ ROM / instability / atrophy / abnormal strength, tone in head, neck, spine, ribs, pelvis, UE, LE / pathologic reflexes

PSYCH — A&O x3 / +recent/remote memory / insight / affect

BREAST — nipple abnormality / mass / tenderness / axillary, clavicular adenopathy

GYN/GU — lesions / d/c / uterus, adnexa tenderness / CMT // circumcised / penile lesions / urethra normal location, no d/c / testes normal / + cremasteric reflex

FEET — + pulses / monofilament + / nails abnormal / dry, broken skin / callus

---

LABS — CBC / CMP / lipids / TSH / microalbumin / A1C / UA, culture / PSA / iron studies / other:

DIAGNOSTICS — XR / MRI / CT / US / cardiac / other

REFERRALS —   **F/U** ___ wk ___ mo

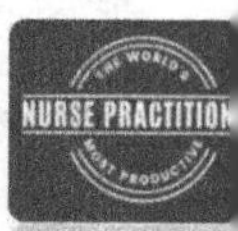

<table>
<tr><td colspan="2">

Patient ID#:

Reason for visit:
</td><td>

Date of visit:

Age: **Gender:**
</td></tr>
</table>

<table>
<tr><td>

BP:

HR:

T:

O2%:
</td><td>

HT:

WT:

BMI:

PAIN:
</td></tr>
</table>

NOTES . . . .

CONST	Δ appetite, energy, weight / fever / chills / sweats / fatigue
HEAD	trauma / mass / tenderness / rash / lesions
EYES	visionΔ / itch / d/c / tears / dry / cataracts / glaucoma / glasses, contacts
ENT	hearing Δ / pain / d/c / vertigo / ? infection // epistaxis / congestion // bleeding, swelling gums / pain / sore throat / voice Δ // neck pain / lumps / swelling / difficulty swallowing
CARDIAC	pain / pressure / dizzy / N / orthopnea / edema / palp / weak w exertion / hx murmurs / hx MI / HTN / HF / numb / tingle / cold extrem / slow wound healing
RESP	wheeze / SOB / cough / asthma / bronch / COPD
GI	abd pain / Δ in bowels / constipation / diarrhea / N V / hepatitis / gallstones / dysphagia / reflux / hemorrhoids / black, bloody stools
GU	burn / pain / nocturia / polyuria / hematuria / incontinence / infection / kid. stones
GENITAL	DC / sores / pain / masses / last pap ______ / sexually active Y N / dyspareunia / LMP ______ / contraception
MSK	redness / swelling / warmth / pain / +/- ROM / arthritis / musc cramps / fracture / sprains / joint replacement / stiffness: AM PM
SKIN	rash / pruritis / jaundice / bruising / hx skin ca / mole Δ / Δ in hair, nails / lesions / slow wound healing
BREASTS	lump / pain / dc / last mammo ______ / self exams YN
NEURO	HA / seizure / vertigo / memory Δ / gait Δ / speech / coord
PSYCH	depression / anxiety / Δ in sleep pattern / substance, ETOH abuse / suicidal ideation / homicidal ideation
ENDO	polydipsia, polyuria / heat, cold intolerance / Δ hair/nails/energy
HEM/LYMPH	anemia / bruising / hx transfusions / blood disorder / lymphadenopathy / axillary, groin tenderness
ALLX/IMMUN	season allx / food allx / med allx / immune disorder:

SOCIAL HX	# in household ______ / lives with SP/BF/GF/SO / children ___ / tobacco Y/N #pk / sexual activity Y/N / etoh, other substances Y/N / occupation:
FAM HX	ca / HTN / MI / CAD / stroke / hyperlipidemia / DM2 / Alzheimer's / depression / osteoporosis / other:

GENERAL	well appearing / well nourished / a&o x 3 / normal mood / normal affect
NEURO	intact / abnormal **DTR:** 1 2 3 4 5 location:
SKIN + NAILS	turgor / rash / bruising / lesions // texture, distribution of hair // nails: abnormal color / nail deformity
HEAD	normocephalic / atraumatic / visible mass / palpable mass / depression / scarring
EYES	acuity intact / conjunctiva clear / EOM intact / PERRLA / fundi: normal discs and vessels / icterus / exudate / hemorrhage
EARS	EACs clear / TM translucent, mobile / landmarks abnormal / hearing diminished
NOSE	lesions / mucosal inflammation / septum, turbinates abnormal / sinus tenderness
MOUTH	mucous membranes dry / lesions / poor dentition / caries / gingival inflammation
PHARYNX	mucosa inflammation / tonsillar hypertrophy / tonsillar exudate
NECK	supple / ROM WNL / lesion / bruit / adenopathy / thyroid enlarged, tender / mass
CARDIAC	regular rate, rhythm / S1, S2 / murmur / gallop / click / rub / PMI displacement
RESP	clear to auscultation in all fields / wheezes (insp) (exp) / rales / crackles
ABDOMEN	BSx4 / tender / organomegaly / mass / hernia
RECTAL	abnormal tone / hemorrhoids (int/ext) / palpable mass
BACK	abnormal curvature / tenderness / CVAT / Δ ROM
EXTREMITIES	amputation / deformity / edema / varicosities / + pulses
MSK	abnormal gait / asymmetry / crepitation / defect / tenderness / mass / effusion / Δ ROM / instability / atrophy / abnormal strength, tone in head, neck, spine, ribs, pelvis, UE, LE / pathologic reflexes
PSYCH	A&O x3 / +recent/remote memory / insight / affect
BREAST	nipple abnormality / mass / tenderness / axillary, clavicular adenopathy
GYN/GU	lesions / d/c / uterus, adnexa tenderness / CMT // circumcised / penile lesions / urethra normal location, no d/c / testes normal / + cremasteric reflex
FEET	+ pulses / monofilament + / nails abnormal / dry, broken skin / callus

LABS	CBC / CMP / lipids / TSH / microalbumin / A1C / UA, culture / PSA / iron studies / other:

DIAGNOSTICS	XR / MRI / CT / US / cardiac / other
REFERRALS	**F/U** ___ wk ___ mo

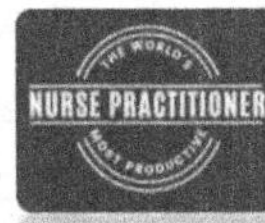

<table>
<tr><td colspan="2">Patient ID#:
Reason for visit:</td><td>Date of visit:
Age:　　Gender:</td></tr>
</table>

BP: 　　　　**HT:**
HR: 　　　　**WT:**
T: 　　　　**BMI:**
O2%: 　　　**PAIN:**

NOTES . . . .

CONST Δ appetite, energy, weight / fever / chills / sweats / fatigue
HEAD trauma / mass / tenderness / rash / lesions
EYES visionΔ / itch / d/c / tears / dry / cataracts / glaucoma / glasses, contacts
ENT hearing Δ / pain / d/c / vertigo / ? infection // epistaxis / congestion // bleeding, swelling gums / pain / sore throat / voice Δ // neck pain / lumps / swelling / difficulty swallowing

CARDIAC pain / pressure / dizzy / N / orthopnea / edema / palp / weak w exertion / hx murmurs / hx MI / HTN / HF / numb / tingle / cold extrem / slow wound healing
RESP wheeze / SOB / cough / asthma / bronch / COPD
GI abd pain / Δ in bowels / constipation / diarrhea / N V / hepatitis / gallstones / dysphagia / reflux / hemorrhoids / black, bloody stools
GU burn / pain / nocturia / polyuria / hematuria / incontinence / infection / kid. stones
GENITAL DC / sores / pain / masses / last pap ______ / sexually active Y N / dyspareunia / LMP ______ / contraception
MSK redness / swelling / warmth / pain / +/- ROM / arthritis / musc cramps / fracture / sprains / joint replacement / stiffness: AM PM
SKIN rash / pruritis / jaundice / bruising / hx skin ca / mole Δ / Δ in hair, nails / lesions / slow wound healing
BREASTS lump / pain / dc / last mammo ______ / self exams YN
NEURO HA / seizure / vertigo / memory Δ / gait Δ / speech / coord
PSYCH depression / anxiety / Δ in sleep pattern / substance, ETOH abuse / suicidal ideation / homicidal ideation
ENDO polydipsia, polyuria / heat, cold intolerance / Δ hair/nails/energy
HEM/LYMPH anemia / bruising / hx transfusions / blood disorder / lymphadenopathy / axillary, groin tenderness
ALLX/IMMUN season allx / food allx / med allx / immune disorder:

SOCIAL HX # in household ______ / lives with SP/BF/GF/SO / children __ / tobacco Y/N #pk / sexual activity Y/N / etoh, other substances Y/N / occupation:
FAM HX ca / HTN / MI / CAD / stroke / hyperlipidemia / DM2 / Alzheimer's / depression / osteoporosis / other:

GENERAL well appearing / well nourished / a&o x 3 / normal mood / normal affect
NEURO intact / abnormal 　　　　　**DTR:** 1 2 3 4 5 location:
SKIN + NAILS turgor / rash / bruising / lesions // texture, distribution of hair // nails: abnormal color / nail deformity
HEAD normocephalic / atraumatic / visible mass / palpable mass / depression / scarring
EYES acuity intact / conjunctiva clear / EOM intact / PERRLA / fundi: normal discs and vessels / icterus / exudate / hemorrhage
EARS EACs clear / TM translucent, mobile / landmarks abnormal / hearing diminished
NOSE lesions / mucosal inflammation / septum, turbinates abnormal / sinus tenderness
MOUTH mucous membranes dry / lesions / poor dentition / caries / gingival inflammation
PHARYNX mucosa inflammation / tonsillar hypertrophy / tonsillar exudate
NECK supple / ROM WNL / lesion / bruit / adenopathy / thyroid enlarged, tender / mass
CARDIAC regular rate, rhythm / S1, S2 / murmur / gallop / click / rub / PMI displacement
RESP clear to auscultation in all fields / wheezes (insp) (exp) / rales / crackles
ABDOMEN BSx4 / tender / organomegaly / mass / hernia
RECTAL abnormal tone / hemorrhoids (int/ext) / palpable mass
BACK abnormal curvature / tenderness / CVAT / Δ ROM
EXTREMITIES amputation / deformity / edema / varicosities / + pulses
MSK abnormal gait / asymmetry / crepitation / defect / tenderness / mass / effusion / Δ ROM / instability / atrophy / abnormal strength, tone in head, neck, spine, ribs, pelvis, UE, LE / pathologic reflexes
PSYCH A&O x3 / +recent/remote memory / insight / affect
BREAST nipple abnormality / mass / tenderness / axillary, clavicular adenopathy
GYN/GU lesions / d/c / uterus, adnexa tenderness / CMT // circumcised / penile lesions / urethra normal location, no d/c / testes normal / + cremasteric reflex
FEET + pulses / monofilament + / nails abnormal / dry, broken skin / callus

LABS CBC / CMP / lipids / TSH / microalbumin / A1C / UA, culture / PSA / iron studies / other:

DIAGNOSTICS XR / MRI / CT / US / cardiac / other
REFERRALS 　　　　　　　**F/U** ___ wk ___ mo

Patient ID#:	Date of visit:		BP:	HT:
Reason for visit:	Age:	Gender:	HR:	WT:
			T:	BMI:
			O2%:	PAIN:

NOTES . . . .

CONST	Δ appetite, energy, weight / fever / chills / sweats / fatigue
HEAD	trauma / mass / tenderness / rash / lesions
EYES	visionΔ / itch / d/c / tears / dry / cataracts / glaucoma / glasses, contacts
ENT	hearing Δ / pain / d/c / vertigo / ? infection // epistaxis / congestion // bleeding, swelling gums / pain / sore throat / voice Δ // neck pain / lumps / swelling / difficulty swallowing
CARDIAC	pain / pressure / dizzy / N / orthopnea / edema / palp / weak w exertion / hx murmurs / hx MI / HTN / HF / numb / tingle / cold extrem / slow wound healing
RESP	wheeze / SOB / cough / asthma / bronch / COPD
GI	abd pain / Δ in bowels / constipation / diarrhea / N V / hepatitis / gallstones / dysphagia / reflux / hemorrhoids / black, bloody stools
GU	burn / pain / nocturia / polyuria / hematuria / incontinence / infection / kid. stones
GENITAL	DC / sores / pain / masses / last pap ______ / sexually active Y N / dyspareunia / LMP ______ / contraception
MSK	redness / swelling / warmth / pain / +/- ROM / arthritis / musc cramps / fracture / sprains / joint replacement / stiffness: AM PM
SKIN	rash / pruritis / jaundice / bruising / hx skin ca / mole Δ / Δ in hair, nails / lesions / slow wound healing
BREASTS	lump / pain / dc / last mammo ______ / self exams YN
NEURO	HA / seizure / vertigo / memory Δ / gait Δ / speech / coord
PSYCH	depression / anxiety / Δ in sleep pattern / substance, ETOH abuse / suicidal ideation / homicidal ideation
ENDO	polydipsia, polyuria / heat, cold intolerance / Δ hair/nails/energy
HEM/LYMPH	anemia / bruising / hx transfusions / blood disorder / lymphadenopathy / axillary, groin tenderness
ALLX/IMMUN	season allx / food allx / med allx / immune disorder:
SOCIAL HX	# in household ______ / lives with SP/BF/GF/SO / children __ / tobacco Y/N #pk / sexual activity Y/N / etoh, other substances Y/N / occupation:
FAM HX	ca / HTN / MI / CAD / stroke / hyperlipidemia / DM2 / Alzheimer's / depression / osteoporosis / other:
GENERAL	well appearing / well nourished / a&o x 3 / normal mood / normal affect
NEURO	intact / abnormal **DTR:** 1 2 3 4 5 location:
SKIN + NAILS	turgor / rash / bruising / lesions // texture, distribution of hair // nails: abnormal color / nail deformity
HEAD	normocephalic / atraumatic / visible mass / palpable mass / depression / scarring
EYES	acuity intact / conjunctiva clear / EOM intact / PERRLA / fundi: normal discs and vessels / icterus / exudate / hemorrhage
EARS	EACs clear / TM translucent, mobile / landmarks abnormal / hearing diminished
NOSE	lesions / mucosal inflammation / septum, turbinates abnormal / sinus tenderness
MOUTH	mucous membranes dry / lesions / poor dentition / caries / gingival inflammation
PHARYNX	mucosa inflammation / tonsillar hypertrophy / tonsillar exudate
NECK	supple / ROM WNL / lesion / bruit / adenopathy / thyroid enlarged, tender / mass
CARDIAC	regular rate, rhythm / S1, S2 / murmur / gallop / click / rub / PMI displacement
RESP	clear to auscultation in all fields / wheezes (insp) (exp) / rales / crackles
ABDOMEN	BSx4 / tender / organomegaly / mass / hernia
RECTAL	abnormal tone / hemorrhoids (int/ext) / palpable mass
BACK	abnormal curvature / tenderness / CVAT / Δ ROM
EXTREMITIES	amputation / deformity / edema / varicosities / + pulses
MSK	abnormal gait / asymmetry / crepitation / defect / tenderness / mass / effusion / Δ ROM / instability / atrophy / abnormal strength, tone in head, neck, spine, ribs, pelvis, UE, LE / pathologic reflexes
PSYCH	A&O x3 / +recent/remote memory / insight / affect
BREAST	nipple abnormality / mass / tenderness / axillary, clavicular adenopathy
GYN/GU	lesions / d/c / uterus, adnexa tenderness / CMT // circumcised / penile lesions / urethra normal location, no d/c / testes normal / + cremasteric reflex
FEET	+ pulses / monofilament + / nails abnormal / dry, broken skin / callus
LABS	CBC / CMP / lipids / TSH / microalbumin / A1C / UA, culture / PSA / iron studies / other:
DIAGNOSTICS	XR / MRI / CT / US / cardiac / other
REFERRALS	**F/U** ___ wk ___ mo

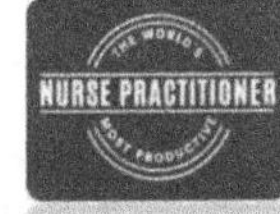

<table>
<tr><td>

Patient ID#:

Reason for visit:
</td><td>

Date of visit:

Age: Gender:
</td></tr>
</table>

BP:	HT:
HR:	WT:
T:	BMI:
O2%:	PAIN:

NOTES . . . .

CONST	Δ appetite, energy, weight / fever / chills / sweats / fatigue
HEAD	trauma / mass / tenderness / rash / lesions
EYES	visionΔ / itch / d/c / tears / dry / cataracts / glaucoma / glasses, contacts
ENT	hearing Δ / pain / d/c / vertigo / ? infection // epistaxis / congestion // bleeding, swelling gums / pain / sore throat / voice Δ // neck pain / lumps / swelling / difficulty swallowing
CARDIAC	pain / pressure / dizzy / N / orthopnea / edema / palp / weak w exertion / hx murmurs / hx MI / HTN / HF / numb / tingle / cold extrem / slow wound healing
RESP	wheeze / SOB / cough / asthma / bronch / COPD
GI	abd pain / Δ in bowels / constipation / diarrhea / N V / hepatitis / gallstones / dysphagia / reflux / hemorrhoids / black, bloody stools
GU	burn / pain / nocturia / polyuria / hematuria / incontinence / infection / kid. stones
GENITAL	DC / sores / pain / masses / last pap _____ / sexually active Y N / dyspareunia / LMP / contraception
MSK	redness / swelling / warmth / pain / +/- ROM / arthritis / musc cramps / fracture / sprains / joint replacement / stiffness: AM PM
SKIN	rash / pruritis / jaundice / bruising / hx skin ca / mole Δ / Δ in hair, nails / lesions / slow wound healing
BREASTS	lump / pain / dc / last mammo / self exams YN
NEURO	HA / seizure / vertigo / memory Δ / gait Δ / speech / coord
PSYCH	depression / anxiety / Δ in sleep pattern / substance, ETOH abuse / suicidal ideation / homicidal ideation
ENDO	polydipsia, polyuria / heat, cold intolerance / Δ hair/nails/energy
HEM/LYMPH	anemia / bruising / hx transfusions / blood disorder / lymphadenopathy / axillary, groin tenderness
ALLX/IMMUN	season allx / food allx / med allx / immune disorder:
SOCIAL HX	# in household _____ / lives with SP/BF/GF/SO / children __ / tobacco Y/N #pk / sexual activity Y/N / etoh, other substances Y/N / occupation:
FAM HX	ca / HTN / MI / CAD / stroke / hyperlipidemia / DM2 / Alzheimer's / depression / osteoporosis / other:
GENERAL	well appearing / well nourished / a&o x 3 / normal mood / normal affect
NEURO	intact / abnormal **DTR:** 1 2 3 4 5 location:
SKIN + NAILS	turgor / rash / bruising / lesions // texture, distribution of hair // nails: abnormal color / nail deformity
HEAD	normocephalic / atraumatic / visible mass / palpable mass / depression / scarring
EYES	acuity intact / conjunctiva clear / EOM intact / PERRLA / fundi: normal discs and vessels / icterus / exudate / hemorrhage
EARS	EACs clear / TM translucent, mobile / landmarks abnormal / hearing diminished
NOSE	lesions / mucosal inflammation / septum, turbinates abnormal / sinus tenderness
MOUTH	mucous membranes dry / lesions / poor dentition / caries / gingival inflammation
PHARYNX	mucosa inflammation / tonsillar hypertrophy / tonsillar exudate
NECK	supple / ROM WNL / lesion / bruit / adenopathy / thyroid enlarged, tender / mass
CARDIAC	regular rate, rhythm / S1, S2 / murmur / gallop / click / rub / PMI displacement
RESP	clear to auscultation in all fields / wheezes (insp) (exp) / rales / crackles
ABDOMEN	BSx4 / tender / organomegaly / mass / hernia
RECTAL	abnormal tone / hemorrhoids (int/ext) / palpable mass
BACK	abnormal curvature / tenderness / CVAT / Δ ROM
EXTREMITIES	amputation / deformity / edema / varicosities / + pulses
MSK	abnormal gait / asymmetry / crepitation / defect / tenderness / mass / effusion / Δ ROM / instability / atrophy / abnormal strength, tone in head, neck, spine, ribs, pelvis, UE, LE / pathologic reflexes
PSYCH	A&O x3 / +recent/remote memory / insight / affect
BREAST	nipple abnormality / mass / tenderness / axillary, clavicular adenopathy
GYN/GU	lesions / d/c / uterus, adnexa tenderness / CMT // circumcised / penile lesions / urethra normal location, no d/c / testes normal / + cremasteric reflex
FEET	+ pulses / monofilament + / nails abnormal / dry, broken skin / callus
LABS	CBC / CMP / lipids / TSH / microalbumin / A1C / UA, culture / PSA / iron studies / other:
DIAGNOSTICS	XR / MRI / CT / US / cardiac / other
REFERRALS	**F/U** ___ wk ___ mo

<table>
<tr><td colspan="2">

Patient ID#:   **Date of visit:**
Reason for visit: **Age:**   **Gender:**

</td><td>

BP: **HT:**
HR: **WT:**
T: **BMI:**
O2%:   **PAIN:**

NOTES . . . .

</td></tr>
</table>

CONST Δ appetite, energy, weight / fever / chills / sweats / fatigue
HEAD trauma / mass / tenderness / rash / lesions
EYES visionΔ / itch / d/c / tears / dry / cataracts / glaucoma / glasses, contacts
ENT hearing Δ / pain / d/c / vertigo / ? infection // epistaxis / congestion // bleeding, swelling gums / pain / sore throat / voice Δ // neck pain / lumps / swelling / difficulty swallowing

CARDIAC pain / pressure / dizzy / N / orthopnea / edema / palp / weak w exertion / hx murmurs / hx MI / HTN / HF / numb / tingle / cold extrem / slow wound healing
RESP wheeze / SOB / cough / asthma / bronch / COPD
GI abd pain / Δ in bowels / constipation / diarrhea / N V / hepatitis / gallstones / dysphagia / reflux / hemorrhoids / black, bloody stools
GU burn / pain / nocturia / polyuria / hematuria / incontinence / infection / kid. stones
GENITAL DC / sores / pain / masses / last pap ______ / sexually active Y N / dyspareunia / LMP ______ / contraception
MSK redness / swelling / warmth / pain / +/- ROM / arthritis / musc cramps / fracture / sprains / joint replacement / stiffness: AM PM
SKIN rash / pruritis / jaundice / bruising / hx skin ca / mole Δ / Δ in hair, nails / lesions / slow wound healing
BREASTS lump / pain / dc / last mammo ______ / self exams YN
NEURO HA / seizure / vertigo / memory Δ / gait Δ / speech / coord
PSYCH depression / anxiety / Δ in sleep pattern / substance, ETOH abuse / suicidal ideation / homicidal ideation
ENDO polydipsia, polyuria / heat, cold intolerance / Δ hair/nails/energy
HEM/LYMPH anemia / bruising / hx transfusions / blood disorder / lymphadenopathy / axillary, groin tenderness
ALLX/IMMUN season allx / food allx / med allx / immune disorder:

SOCIAL HX # in household ______ / lives with SP/BF/GF/SO / children __ / tobacco Y/N #pk / sexual activity Y/N / etoh, other substances Y/N / occupation:
FAM HX ca / HTN / MI / CAD / stroke / hyperlipidemia / DM2 / Alzheimer's / depression / osteoporosis / other:

GENERAL well appearing / well nourished / a&o x 3 / normal mood / normal affect
NEURO intact / abnormal   **DTR:** 1 2 3 4 5 location:
SKIN + NAILS turgor / rash / bruising / lesions // texture, distribution of hair // nails: abnormal color / nail deformity
HEAD normocephalic / atraumatic / visible mass / palpable mass / depression / scarring
EYES acuity intact / conjunctiva clear / EOM intact / PERRLA / fundi: normal discs and vessels / icterus / exudate / hemorrhage
EARS EACs clear / TM translucent, mobile / landmarks abnormal / hearing diminished
NOSE lesions / mucosal inflammation / septum, turbinates abnormal / sinus tenderness
MOUTH mucous membranes dry / lesions / poor dentition / caries / gingival inflammation
PHARYNX mucosa inflammation / tonsillar hypertrophy / tonsillar exudate
NECK supple / ROM WNL / lesion / bruit / adenopathy / thyroid enlarged, tender / mass
CARDIAC regular rate, rhythm / S1, S2 / murmur / gallop / click / rub / PMI displacement
RESP clear to auscultation in all fields / wheezes (insp) (exp) / rales / crackles
ABDOMEN BSx4 / tender / organomegaly / mass / hernia
RECTAL abnormal tone / hemorrhoids (int/ext) / palpable mass
BACK abnormal curvature / tenderness / CVAT / Δ ROM
EXTREMITIES amputation / deformity / edema / varicosities / + pulses
MSK abnormal gait / asymmetry / crepitation / defect / tenderness / mass / effusion / Δ ROM / instability / atrophy / abnormal strength, tone in head, neck, spine, ribs, pelvis, UE, LE / pathologic reflexes
PSYCH A&O x3 / +recent/remote memory / insight / affect
BREAST nipple abnormality / mass / tenderness / axillary, clavicular adenopathy
GYN/GU lesions / d/c / uterus, adnexa tenderness / CMT // circumcised / penile lesions / urethra normal location, no d/c / testes normal / + cremasteric reflex
FEET + pulses / monofilament + / nails abnormal / dry, broken skin / callus

LABS CBC / CMP / lipids / TSH / microalbumin / A1C / UA, culture / PSA / iron studies / other:

DIAGNOSTICS XR / MRI / CT / US / cardiac / other
REFERRALS   **F/U** ___ wk ___ mo

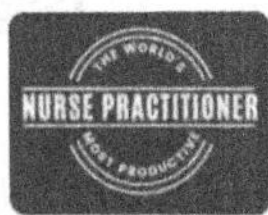

<table>
<tr><td colspan="2">

Patient ID#:   **Date of visit:**
Reason for visit: **Age:**   **Gender:**

</td><td>

BP: **HT:**
HR: **WT:**
T: **BMI:**
O2%:   **PAIN:**

</td></tr>
</table>

NOTES . . . .

CONST	Δ appetite, energy, weight / fever / chills / sweats / fatigue
HEAD	trauma / mass / tenderness / rash / lesions
EYES	visionΔ / itch / d/c / tears / dry / cataracts / glaucoma / glasses, contacts
ENT	hearing Δ / pain / d/c / vertigo / ? infection // epistaxis / congestion // bleeding, swelling gums / pain / sore throat / voice Δ // neck pain / lumps / swelling / difficulty swallowing
CARDIAC	pain / pressure / dizzy / N / orthopnea / edema / palp / weak w exertion / hx murmurs / hx MI / HTN / HF / numb / tingle / cold extrem / slow wound healing
RESP	wheeze / SOB / cough / asthma / bronch / COPD
GI	abd pain / Δ in bowels / constipation / diarrhea / N V / hepatitis / gallstones / dysphagia / reflux / hemorrhoids / black, bloody stools
GU	burn / pain / nocturia / polyuria / hematuria / incontinence / infection / kid. stones
GENITAL	DC / sores / pain / masses / last pap _____ / sexually active Y N / dyspareunia / LMP _____ / contraception
MSK	redness / swelling / warmth / pain / +/- ROM / arthritis / musc cramps / fracture / sprains / joint replacement / stiffness: AM PM
SKIN	rash / pruritis / jaundice / bruising / hx skin ca / mole Δ / Δ in hair, nails / lesions / slow wound healing
BREASTS	lump / pain / dc / last mammo _____ / self exams YN
NEURO	HA / seizure / vertigo / memory Δ / gait Δ / speech / coord
PSYCH	depression / anxiety / Δ in sleep pattern / substance, ETOH abuse / suicidal ideation / homicidal ideation
ENDO	polydipsia, polyuria / heat, cold intolerance / Δ hair/nails/energy
HEM/LYMPH	anemia / bruising / hx transfusions / blood disorder / lymphadenopathy / axillary, groin tenderness
ALLX/IMMUN	season allx / food allx / med allx / immune disorder:
SOCIAL HX	# in household _____ / lives with SP/BF/GF/SO / children __ / tobacco Y/N #pk / sexual activity Y/N / etoh, other substances Y/N / occupation:
FAM HX	ca / HTN / MI / CAD / stroke / hyperlipidemia / DM2 / Alzheimer's / depression / osteoporosis / other:
GENERAL	well appearing / well nourished / a&o x 3 / normal mood / normal affect
NEURO	intact / abnormal **DTR:** 1 2 3 4 5 location:
SKIN + NAILS	turgor / rash / bruising / lesions // texture, distribution of hair // nails: abnormal color / nail deformity
HEAD	normocephalic / atraumatic / visible mass / palpable mass / depression / scarring
EYES	acuity intact / conjunctiva clear / EOM intact / PERRLA / fundi: normal discs and vessels / icterus / exudate / hemorrhage
EARS	EACs clear / TM translucent, mobile / landmarks abnormal / hearing diminished
NOSE	lesions / mucosal inflammation / septum, turbinates abnormal / sinus tenderness
MOUTH	mucous membranes dry / lesions / poor dentition / caries / gingival inflammation
PHARYNX	mucosa inflammation / tonsillar hypertrophy / tonsillar exudate
NECK	supple / ROM WNL / lesion / bruit / adenopathy / thyroid enlarged, tender / mass
CARDIAC	regular rate, rhythm / S1, S2 / murmur / gallop / click / rub / PMI displacement
RESP	clear to auscultation in all fields / wheezes (insp) (exp) / rales / crackles
ABDOMEN	BSx4 / tender / organomegaly / mass / hernia
RECTAL	abnormal tone / hemorrhoids (int/ext) / palpable mass
BACK	abnormal curvature / tenderness / CVAT / Δ ROM
EXTREMITIES	amputation / deformity / edema / varicosities / + pulses
MSK	abnormal gait / asymmetry / crepitation / defect / tenderness / mass / effusion / Δ ROM / instability / atrophy / abnormal strength, tone in head, neck, spine, ribs, pelvis, UE, LE / pathologic reflexes
PSYCH	A&O x3 / +recent/remote memory / insight / affect
BREAST	nipple abnormality / mass / tenderness / axillary, clavicular adenopathy
GYN/GU	lesions / d/c / uterus, adnexa tenderness / CMT // circumcised / penile lesions / urethra normal location, no d/c / testes normal / + cremasteric reflex
FEET	+ pulses / monofilament + / nails abnormal / dry, broken skin / callus
LABS	CBC / CMP / lipids / TSH / microalbumin / A1C / UA, culture / PSA / iron studies / other:
DIAGNOSTICS	XR / MRI / CT / US / cardiac / other
REFERRALS	**F/U** ___ wk ___ mo

<table>
<tr><td>Patient ID#:</td><td>Date of visit:</td></tr>
<tr><td>Reason for visit:</td><td>Age: Gender:</td></tr>
</table>

BP:	HT:
HR:	WT:
T:	BMI:
O2%:	PAIN:

NOTES . . . .

CONST	Δ appetite, energy, weight / fever / chills / sweats / fatigue
HEAD	trauma / mass / tenderness / rash / lesions
EYES	visionΔ / itch / d/c / tears / dry / cataracts / glaucoma / glasses, contacts
ENT	hearing Δ / pain / d/c / vertigo / ? infection // epistaxis / congestion // bleeding, swelling gums / pain / sore throat / voice Δ // neck pain / lumps / swelling / difficulty swallowing
CARDIAC	pain / pressure / dizzy / N / orthopnea / edema / palp / weak w exertion / hx murmurs / hx MI / HTN / HF / numb / tingle / cold extrem / slow wound healing
RESP	wheeze / SOB / cough / asthma / bronch / COPD
GI	abd pain / Δ in bowels / constipation / diarrhea / N V / hepatitis / gallstones / dysphagia / reflux / hemorrhoids / black, bloody stools
GU	burn / pain / nocturia / polyuria / hematuria / incontinence / infection / kid. stones
GENITAL	DC / sores / pain / masses / last pap ______ / sexually active Y N / dyspareunia / LMP ______ / contraception
MSK	redness / swelling / warmth / pain / +/- ROM / arthritis / musc cramps / fracture / sprains / joint replacement / stiffness: AM PM
SKIN	rash / pruritis / jaundice / bruising / hx skin ca / mole Δ / Δ in hair, nails / lesions / slow wound healing
BREASTS	lump / pain / dc / last mammo ______ / self exams YN
NEURO	HA / seizure / vertigo / memory Δ / gait Δ / speech / coord
PSYCH	depression / anxiety / Δ in sleep pattern / substance, ETOH abuse / suicidal ideation / homicidal ideation
ENDO	polydipsia, polyuria / heat, cold intolerance / Δ hair/nails/energy
HEM/LYMPH	anemia / bruising / hx transfusions / blood disorder / lymphadenopathy / axillary, groin tenderness
ALLX/IMMUN	season allx / food allx / med allx / immune disorder:
SOCIAL HX	# in household ______ / lives with SP/BF/GF/SO / children __ / tobacco Y/N #pk / sexual activity Y/N / etoh, other substances Y/N / occupation:
FAM HX	ca / HTN / MI / CAD / stroke / hyperlipidemia / DM2 / Alzheimer's / depression / osteoporosis / other:
GENERAL	well appearing / well nourished / a&o x 3 / normal mood / normal affect
NEURO	intact / abnormal **DTR:** 1 2 3 4 5 location:
SKIN + NAILS	turgor / rash / bruising / lesions // texture, distribution of hair // nails: abnormal color / nail deformity
HEAD	normocephalic / atraumatic / visible mass / palpable mass / depression / scarring
EYES	acuity intact / conjunctiva clear / EOM intact / PERRLA / fundi: normal discs and vessels / icterus / exudate / hemorrhage
EARS	EACs clear / TM translucent, mobile / landmarks abnormal / hearing diminished
NOSE	lesions / mucosal inflammation / septum, turbinates abnormal / sinus tenderness
MOUTH	mucous membranes dry / lesions / poor dentition / caries / gingival inflammation
PHARYNX	mucosa inflammation / tonsillar hypertrophy / tonsillar exudate
NECK	supple / ROM WNL / lesion / bruit / adenopathy / thyroid enlarged, tender / mass
CARDIAC	regular rate, rhythm / S1, S2 / murmur / gallop / click / rub / PMI displacement
RESP	clear to auscultation in all fields / wheezes (insp) (exp) / rales / crackles
ABDOMEN	BSx4 / tender / organomegaly / mass / hernia
RECTAL	abnormal tone / hemorrhoids (int/ext) / palpable mass
BACK	abnormal curvature / tenderness / CVAT / Δ ROM
EXTREMITIES	amputation / deformity / edema / varicosities / + pulses
MSK	abnormal gait / asymmetry / crepitation / defect / tenderness / mass / effusion / Δ ROM / instability / atrophy / abnormal strength, tone in head, neck, spine, ribs, pelvis, UE, LE / pathologic reflexes
PSYCH	A&O x3 / +recent/remote memory / insight / affect
BREAST	nipple abnormality / mass / tenderness / axillary, clavicular adenopathy
GYN/GU	lesions / d/c / uterus, adnexa tenderness / CMT // circumcised / penile lesions / urethra normal location, no d/c / testes normal / + cremasteric reflex
FEET	+ pulses / monofilament + / nails abnormal / dry, broken skin / callus
LABS	CBC / CMP / lipids / TSH / microalbumin / A1C / UA, culture / PSA / iron studies / other:
DIAGNOSTICS	XR / MRI / CT / US / cardiac / other
REFERRALS	**F/U** ___ wk ___ mo

<table>
<tr><td>Patient ID#:</td><td>Date of visit:</td></tr>
<tr><td>Reason for visit:</td><td>Age: Gender:</td></tr>
</table>

NOTES . . . .

CONST Δ appetite, energy, weight / fever / chills / sweats / fatigue

HEAD trauma / mass / tenderness / rash / lesions

EYES visionΔ / itch / d/c / tears / dry / cataracts / glaucoma / glasses, contacts

ENT hearing Δ / pain / d/c / vertigo / ? infection // epistaxis / congestion // bleeding, swelling gums / pain / sore throat / voice Δ // neck pain / lumps / swelling / difficulty swallowing

CARDIAC pain / pressure / dizzy / N / orthopnea / edema / palp / weak w exertion / hx murmurs / hx MI / HTN / HF / numb / tingle / cold extrem / slow wound healing

RESP wheeze / SOB / cough / asthma / bronch / COPD

GI abd pain / Δ in bowels / constipation / diarrhea / N V / hepatitis / gallstones / dysphagia / reflux / hemorrhoids / black, bloody stools

GU burn / pain / nocturia / polyuria / hematuria / incontinence / infection / kid. stones

GENITAL DC / sores / pain / masses / last pap ______ / sexually active Y N / dyspareunia / LMP ________ / contraception

MSK redness / swelling / warmth / pain / +/- ROM / arthritis / musc cramps / fracture / sprains / joint replacement / stiffness: AM PM

SKIN rash / pruritis / jaundice / bruising / hx skin ca / mole Δ / Δ in hair, nails / lesions / slow wound healing

BREASTS lump / pain / dc / last mammo ______ / self exams YN

NEURO HA / seizure / vertigo / memory Δ / gait Δ / speech / coord

PSYCH depression / anxiety / Δ in sleep pattern / substance, ETOH abuse / suicidal ideation / homicidal ideation

ENDO polydipsia, polyuria / heat, cold intolerance / Δ hair/nails/energy

HEM/LYMPH anemia / bruising / hx transfusions / blood disorder / lymphadenopathy / axillary, groin tenderness

ALLX/IMMUN season allx / food allx / med allx / immune disorder:

SOCIAL HX # in household ______ / lives with SP/BF/GF/SO / children __ / tobacco Y/N #pk / sexual activity Y/N / etoh, other substances Y/N / occupation:

FAM HX ca / HTN / MI / CAD / stroke / hyperlipidemia / DM2 / Alzheimer's / depression / osteoporosis / other:

GENERAL well appearing / well nourished / a&o x 3 / normal mood / normal affect

NEURO intact / abnormal   **DTR:** 1 2 3 4 5 location:

SKIN + NAILS turgor / rash / bruising / lesions // texture, distribution of hair // nails: abnormal color / nail deformity

HEAD normocephalic / atraumatic / visible mass / palpable mass / depression / scarring

EYES acuity intact / conjunctiva clear / EOM intact / PERRLA / fundi: normal discs and vessels / icterus / exudate / hemorrhage

EARS EACs clear / TM translucent, mobile / landmarks abnormal / hearing diminished

NOSE lesions / mucosal inflammation / septum, turbinates abnormal / sinus tenderness

MOUTH mucous membranes dry / lesions / poor dentition / caries / gingival inflammation

PHARYNX mucosa inflammation / tonsillar hypertrophy / tonsillar exudate

NECK supple / ROM WNL / lesion / bruit / adenopathy / thyroid enlarged, tender / mass

CARDIAC regular rate, rhythm / S1, S2 / murmur / gallop / click / rub / PMI displacement

RESP clear to auscultation in all fields / wheezes (insp) (exp) / rales / crackles

ABDOMEN BSx4 / tender / organomegaly / mass / hernia

RECTAL abnormal tone / hemorrhoids (int/ext) / palpable mass

BACK abnormal curvature / tenderness / CVAT / Δ ROM

EXTREMITIES amputation / deformity / edema / varicosities / + pulses

MSK abnormal gait / asymmetry / crepitation / defect / tenderness / mass / effusion / Δ ROM / instability / atrophy / abnormal strength, tone in head, neck, spine, ribs, pelvis, UE, LE / pathologic reflexes

PSYCH A&O x3 / +recent/remote memory / insight / affect

BREAST nipple abnormality / mass / tenderness / axillary, clavicular adenopathy

GYN/GU lesions / d/c / uterus, adnexa tenderness / CMT // circumcised / penile lesions / urethra normal location, no d/c / testes normal / + cremasteric reflex

FEET + pulses / monofilament + / nails abnormal / dry, broken skin / callus

---

LABS CBC / CMP / lipids / TSH / microalbumin / A1C / UA, culture / PSA / iron studies / other:

DIAGNOSTICS XR / MRI / CT / US / cardiac / other

REFERRALS

F/U ___ wk ___ mo

<table>
<tr><td>

Patient ID#:   **Date of visit:**

Reason for visit: **Age:**   **Gender:**

</td><td>

BP: **HT:**
HR: **WT:**
T: **BMI:**
O2%:   **PAIN:**

NOTES . . . .

</td></tr>
</table>

CONST — Δ appetite, energy, weight / fever / chills / sweats / fatigue

HEAD — trauma / mass / tenderness / rash / lesions

EYES — visionΔ / itch / d/c / tears / dry / cataracts / glaucoma / glasses, contacts

ENT — hearing Δ / pain / d/c / vertigo / ? infection // epistaxis / congestion // bleeding, swelling gums / pain / sore throat / voice Δ // neck pain / lumps / swelling / difficulty swallowing

CARDIAC — pain / pressure / dizzy / N / orthopnea / edema / palp / weak w exertion / hx murmurs / hx MI / HTN / HF / numb / tingle / cold extrem / slow wound healing

RESP — wheeze / SOB / cough / asthma / bronch / COPD

GI — abd pain / Δ in bowels / constipation / diarrhea / N V / hepatitis / gallstones / dysphagia / reflux / hemorrhoids / black, bloody stools

GU — burn / pain / nocturia / polyuria / hematuria / incontinence / infection / kid. stones

GENITAL — DC / sores / pain / masses / last pap ______ / sexually active Y N / dyspareunia / LMP ______ / contraception

MSK — redness / swelling / warmth / pain / +/- ROM / arthritis / musc cramps / fracture / sprains / joint replacement / stiffness: AM PM

SKIN — rash / pruritis / jaundice / bruising / hx skin ca / mole Δ / Δ in hair, nails / lesions / slow wound healing

BREASTS — lump / pain / dc / last mammo ______ / self exams YN

NEURO — HA / seizure / vertigo / memory Δ / gait Δ / speech / coord

PSYCH — depression / anxiety / Δ in sleep pattern / substance, ETOH abuse / suicidal ideation / homicidal ideation

ENDO — polydipsia, polyuria / heat, cold intolerance / Δ hair/nails/energy

HEM/LYMPH — anemia / bruising / hx transfusions / blood disorder / lymphadenopathy / axillary, groin tenderness

ALLX/IMMUN — season allx / food allx / med allx / immune disorder:

SOCIAL HX — # in household ______ / lives with SP/BF/GF/SO / children __ / tobacco Y/N #pk / sexual activity Y/N / etoh, other substances Y/N / occupation:

FAM HX — ca / HTN / MI / CAD / stroke / hyperlipidemia / DM2 / Alzheimer's / depression / osteoporosis / other:

GENERAL — well appearing / well nourished / a&o x 3 / normal mood / normal affect

NEURO — intact / abnormal   **DTR:** 1 2 3 4 5 location:

SKIN + NAILS — turgor / rash / bruising / lesions // texture, distribution of hair // nails: abnormal color / nail deformity

HEAD — normocephalic / atraumatic / visible mass / palpable mass / depression / scarring

EYES — acuity intact / conjunctiva clear / EOM intact / PERRLA / fundi: normal discs and vessels / icterus / exudate / hemorrhage

EARS — EACs clear / TM translucent, mobile / landmarks abnormal / hearing diminished

NOSE — lesions / mucosal inflammation / septum, turbinates abnormal / sinus tenderness

MOUTH — mucous membranes dry / lesions / poor dentition / caries / gingival inflammation

PHARYNX — mucosa inflammation / tonsillar hypertrophy / tonsillar exudate

NECK — supple / ROM WNL / lesion / bruit / adenopathy / thyroid enlarged, tender / mass

CARDIAC — regular rate, rhythm / S1, S2 / murmur / gallop / click / rub / PMI displacement

RESP — clear to auscultation in all fields / wheezes (insp) (exp) / rales / crackles

ABDOMEN — BSx4 / tender / organomegaly / mass / hernia

RECTAL — abnormal tone / hemorrhoids (int/ext) / palpable mass

BACK — abnormal curvature / tenderness / CVAT / Δ ROM

EXTREMITIES — amputation / deformity / edema / varicosities / + pulses

MSK — abnormal gait / asymmetry / crepitation / defect / tenderness / mass / effusion / Δ ROM / instability / atrophy / abnormal strength, tone in head, neck, spine, ribs, pelvis, UE, LE / pathologic reflexes

PSYCH — A&O x3 / +recent/remote memory / insight / affect

BREAST — nipple abnormality / mass / tenderness / axillary, clavicular adenopathy

GYN/GU — lesions / d/c / uterus, adnexa tenderness / CMT // circumcised / penile lesions / urethra normal location, no d/c / testes normal / + cremasteric reflex

FEET — + pulses / monofilament + / nails abnormal / dry, broken skin / callus

---

LABS — CBC / CMP / lipids / TSH / microalbumin / A1C / UA, culture / PSA / iron studies / other:

DIAGNOSTICS — XR / MRI / CT / US / cardiac / other

REFERRALS —   **F/U** ___ wk ___ mo

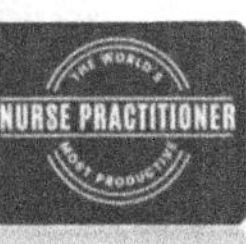

<table>
<tr><td>Patient ID#:
Reason for visit:</td><td>Date of visit:
Age: Gender:</td></tr>
</table>

BP: HT:
HR: WT:
T: BMI:
O2%:   PAIN:

NOTES . . . .

CONST Δ appetite, energy, weight / fever / chills / sweats / fatigue
HEAD trauma / mass / tenderness / rash / lesions
EYES visionΔ / itch / d/c / tears / dry / cataracts / glaucoma / glasses, contacts
ENT hearing Δ / pain / d/c / vertigo / ? infection // epistaxis / congestion // bleeding, swelling gums / pain / sore throat / voice Δ // neck pain / lumps / swelling / difficulty swallowing

CARDIAC pain / pressure / dizzy / N / orthopnea / edema / palp / weak w exertion / hx murmurs / hx MI / HTN / HF / numb / tingle / cold extrem / slow wound healing

RESP wheeze / SOB / cough / asthma / bronch / COPD
GI abd pain / Δ in bowels / constipation / diarrhea / N V / hepatitis / gallstones / dysphagia / reflux / hemorrhoids / black, bloody stools

GU burn / pain / nocturia / polyuria / hematuria / incontinence / infection / kid. stones
GENITAL DC / sores / pain / masses / last pap _____ / sexually active Y N / dyspareunia / LMP _______ / contraception

MSK redness / swelling / warmth / pain / +/- ROM / arthritis / musc cramps / fracture / sprains / joint replacement / stiffness: AM PM

SKIN rash / pruritis / jaundice / bruising / hx skin ca / mole Δ / Δ in hair, nails / lesions / slow wound healing

BREASTS lump / pain / dc / last mammo _______ / self exams YN
NEURO HA / seizure / vertigo / memory Δ / gait Δ / speech / coord
PSYCH depression / anxiety / Δ in sleep pattern / substance, ETOH abuse / suicidal ideation / homicidal ideation

ENDO polydipsia, polyuria / heat, cold intolerance / Δ hair/nails/energy
HEM/LYMPH anemia / bruising / hx transfusions / blood disorder / lymphadenopathy / axillary, groin tenderness

ALLX/IMMUN season allx / food allx / med allx / immune disorder:

SOCIAL HX # in household _____ / lives with SP/BF/GF/SO / children __ / tobacco Y/N #pk / sexual activity Y/N / etoh, other substances Y/N / occupation:
FAM HX ca / HTN / MI / CAD / stroke / hyperlipidemia / DM2 / Alzheimer's / depression / osteoporosis / other:

GENERAL well appearing / well nourished / a&o x 3 / normal mood / normal affect
NEURO intact / abnormal   **DTR:** 1 2 3 4 5 location:
SKIN + NAILS turgor / rash / bruising / lesions // texture, distribution of hair // nails: abnormal color / nail deformity

HEAD normocephalic / atraumatic / visible mass / palpable mass / depression / scarring
EYES acuity intact / conjunctiva clear / EOM intact / PERRLA / fundi: normal discs and vessels / icterus / exudate / hemorrhage

EARS EACs clear / TM translucent, mobile / landmarks abnormal / hearing diminished
NOSE lesions / mucosal inflammation / septum, turbinates abnormal / sinus tenderness
MOUTH mucous membranes dry / lesions / poor dentition / caries / gingival inflammation
PHARYNX mucosa inflammation / tonsillar hypertrophy / tonsillar exudate
NECK supple / ROM WNL / lesion / bruit / adenopathy / thyroid enlarged, tender / mass
CARDIAC regular rate, rhythm / S1, S2 / murmur / gallop / click / rub / PMI displacement
RESP clear to auscultation in all fields / wheezes (insp) (exp) / rales / crackles
ABDOMEN BSx4 / tender / organomegaly / mass / hernia
RECTAL abnormal tone / hemorrhoids (int/ext) / palpable mass
BACK abnormal curvature / tenderness / CVAT / Δ ROM
EXTREMITIES amputation / deformity / edema / varicosities / + pulses
MSK abnormal gait / asymmetry / crepitation / defect / tenderness / mass / effusion / Δ ROM / instability / atrophy / abnormal strength, tone in head, neck, spine, ribs, pelvis, UE, LE / pathologic reflexes

PSYCH A&O x3 / +recent/remote memory / insight / affect
BREAST nipple abnormality / mass / tenderness / axillary, clavicular adenopathy
GYN/GU lesions / d/c / uterus, adnexa tenderness / CMT // circumcised / penile lesions / urethra normal location, no d/c / testes normal / + cremasteric reflex
FEET + pulses / monofilament + / nails abnormal / dry, broken skin / callus

---

LABS CBC / CMP / lipids / TSH / microalbumin / A1C / UA, culture / PSA / iron studies / other:

DIAGNOSTICS XR / MRI / CT / US / cardiac / other
REFERRALS **F/U** ___ wk ___ mo

| Patient ID#: | Date of visit: |
| Reason for visit: | Age: Gender: |

BP: **HT:**
HR: **WT:**
T: **BMI:**
O2%: **PAIN:**

NOTES . . . .

CONST	Δ appetite, energy, weight / fever / chills / sweats / fatigue
HEAD	trauma / mass / tenderness / rash / lesions
EYES	visionΔ / itch / d/c / tears / dry / cataracts / glaucoma / glasses, contacts
ENT	hearing Δ / pain / d/c / vertigo / ? infection // epistaxis / congestion // bleeding, swelling gums / pain / sore throat / voice Δ // neck pain / lumps / swelling / difficulty swallowing
CARDIAC	pain / pressure / dizzy / N / orthopnea / edema / palp / weak w exertion / hx murmurs / hx MI / HTN / HF / numb / tingle / cold extrem / slow wound healing
RESP	wheeze / SOB / cough / asthma / bronch / COPD
GI	abd pain / Δ in bowels / constipation / diarrhea / N V / hepatitis / gallstones / dysphagia / reflux / hemorrhoids / black, bloody stools
GU	burn / pain / nocturia / polyuria / hematuria / incontinence / infection / kid. stones
GENITAL	DC / sores / pain / masses / last pap _____ / sexually active Y N / dyspareunia / LMP _____ / contraception
MSK	redness / swelling / warmth / pain / +/- ROM / arthritis / musc cramps / fracture / sprains / joint replacement / stiffness: AM PM
SKIN	rash / pruritis / jaundice / bruising / hx skin ca / mole Δ / Δ in hair, nails / lesions / slow wound healing
BREASTS	lump / pain / dc / last mammo _____ / self exams YN
NEURO	HA / seizure / vertigo / memory Δ / gait Δ / speech / coord
PSYCH	depression / anxiety / Δ in sleep pattern / substance, ETOH abuse / suicidal ideation / homicidal ideation
ENDO	polydipsia, polyuria / heat, cold intolerance / Δ hair/nails/energy
HEM/LYMPH	anemia / bruising / hx transfusions / blood disorder / lymphadenopathy / axillary, groin tenderness
ALLX/IMMUN	season allx / food allx / med allx / immune disorder:

SOCIAL HX	# in household _____ / lives with SP/BF/GF/SO / children __ / tobacco Y/N #pk / sexual activity Y/N / etoh, other substances Y/N / occupation:
FAM HX	ca / HTN / MI / CAD / stroke / hyperlipidemia / DM2 / Alzheimer's / depression / osteoporosis / other:

GENERAL	well appearing / well nourished / a&o x 3 / normal mood / normal affect
NEURO	intact / abnormal **DTR:** 1 2 3 4 5 location:
SKIN + NAILS	turgor / rash / bruising / lesions // texture, distribution of hair // nails: abnormal color / nail deformity
HEAD	normocephalic / atraumatic / visible mass / palpable mass / depression / scarring
EYES	acuity intact / conjunctiva clear / EOM intact / PERRLA / fundi: normal discs and vessels / icterus / exudate / hemorrhage
EARS	EACs clear / TM translucent, mobile / landmarks abnormal / hearing diminished
NOSE	lesions / mucosal inflammation / septum, turbinates abnormal / sinus tenderness
MOUTH	mucous membranes dry / lesions / poor dentition / caries / gingival inflammation
PHARYNX	mucosa inflammation / tonsillar hypertrophy / tonsillar exudate
NECK	supple / ROM WNL / lesion / bruit / adenopathy / thyroid enlarged, tender / mass
CARDIAC	regular rate, rhythm / S1, S2 / murmur / gallop / click / rub / PMI displacement
RESP	clear to auscultation in all fields / wheezes (insp) (exp) / rales / crackles
ABDOMEN	BSx4 / tender / organomegaly / mass / hernia
RECTAL	abnormal tone / hemorrhoids (int/ext) / palpable mass
BACK	abnormal curvature / tenderness / CVAT / Δ ROM
EXTREMITIES	amputation / deformity / edema / varicosities / + pulses
MSK	abnormal gait / asymmetry / crepitation / defect / tenderness / mass / effusion / Δ ROM / instability / atrophy / abnormal strength, tone in head, neck, spine, ribs, pelvis, UE, LE / pathologic reflexes
PSYCH	A&O x3 / +recent/remote memory / insight / affect
BREAST	nipple abnormality / mass / tenderness / axillary, clavicular adenopathy
GYN/GU	lesions / d/c / uterus, adnexa tenderness / CMT // circumcised / penile lesions / urethra normal location, no d/c / testes normal / + cremasteric reflex
FEET	+ pulses / monofilament + / nails abnormal / dry, broken skin / callus

LABS	CBC / CMP / lipids / TSH / microalbumin / A1C / UA, culture / PSA / iron studies / other:

DIAGNOSTICS	XR / MRI / CT / US / cardiac / other
REFERRALS	**F/U** ___ wk ___ mo

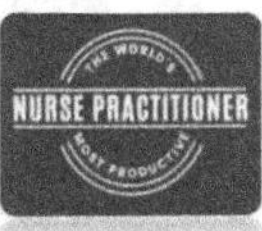

| Patient ID#: | Date of visit: |
| Reason for visit: | Age: Gender: |

BP: HT:
HR: WT:
T: BMI:
O2%:   PAIN:

NOTES . . . .

CONST Δ appetite, energy, weight / fever / chills / sweats / fatigue
HEAD trauma / mass / tenderness / rash / lesions
EYES visionΔ / itch / d/c / tears / dry / cataracts / glaucoma / glasses, contacts
ENT hearing Δ / pain / d/c / vertigo / ? infection // epistaxis / congestion // bleeding, swelling gums / pain / sore throat / voice Δ // neck pain / lumps / swelling / difficulty swallowing

CARDIAC pain / pressure / dizzy / N / orthopnea / edema / palp / weak w exertion / hx murmurs / hx MI / HTN / HF / numb / tingle / cold extrem / slow wound healing

RESP wheeze / SOB / cough / asthma / bronch / COPD
GI abd pain / Δ in bowels / constipation / diarrhea / N V / hepatitis / gallstones / dysphagia / reflux / hemorrhoids / black, bloody stools

GU burn / pain / nocturia / polyuria / hematuria / incontinence / infection / kid. stones
GENITAL DC / sores / pain / masses / last pap ______ / sexually active Y N / dyspareunia / LMP ______ / contraception

MSK redness / swelling / warmth / pain / +/- ROM / arthritis / musc cramps / fracture / sprains / joint replacement / stiffness: AM PM

SKIN rash / pruritis / jaundice / bruising / hx skin ca / mole Δ / Δ in hair, nails / lesions / slow wound healing

BREASTS lump / pain / dc / last mammo ______ / self exams YN
NEURO HA / seizure / vertigo / memory Δ / gait Δ / speech / coord
PSYCH depression / anxiety / Δ in sleep pattern / substance, ETOH abuse / suicidal ideation / homicidal ideation

ENDO polydipsia, polyuria / heat, cold intolerance / Δ hair/nails/energy
HEM/LYMPH anemia / bruising / hx transfusions / blood disorder / lymphadenopathy / axillary, groin tenderness
ALLX/IMMUN season allx / food allx / med allx / immune disorder:

SOCIAL HX # in household ______ / lives with SP/BF/GF/SO / children __ / tobacco Y/N #pk / sexual activity Y/N / etoh, other substances Y/N / occupation:
FAM HX ca / HTN / MI / CAD / stroke / hyperlipidemia / DM2 / Alzheimer's / depression / osteoporosis / other:

GENERAL well appearing / well nourished / a&o x 3 / normal mood / normal affect
NEURO intact / abnormal   **DTR:** 1 2 3 4 5 location:
SKIN + NAILS turgor / rash / bruising / lesions // texture, distribution of hair // nails: abnormal color / nail deformity

HEAD normocephalic / atraumatic / visible mass / palpable mass / depression / scarring
EYES acuity intact / conjunctiva clear / EOM intact / PERRLA / fundi: normal discs and vessels / icterus / exudate / hemorrhage

EARS EACs clear / TM translucent, mobile / landmarks abnormal / hearing diminished
NOSE lesions / mucosal inflammation / septum, turbinates abnormal / sinus tenderness
MOUTH mucous membranes dry / lesions / poor dentition / caries / gingival inflammation
PHARYNX mucosa inflammation / tonsillar hypertrophy / tonsillar exudate
NECK supple / ROM WNL / lesion / bruit / adenopathy / thyroid enlarged, tender / mass
CARDIAC regular rate, rhythm / S1, S2 / murmur / gallop / click / rub / PMI displacement
RESP clear to auscultation in all fields / wheezes (insp) (exp) / rales / crackles
ABDOMEN BSx4 / tender / organomegaly / mass / hernia
RECTAL abnormal tone / hemorrhoids (int/ext) / palpable mass
BACK abnormal curvature / tenderness / CVAT / Δ ROM
EXTREMITIES amputation / deformity / edema / varicosities / + pulses
MSK abnormal gait / asymmetry / crepitation / defect / tenderness / mass / effusion / Δ ROM / instability / atrophy / abnormal strength, tone in head, neck, spine, ribs, pelvis, UE, LE / pathologic reflexes

PSYCH A&O x3 / +recent/remote memory / insight / affect
BREAST nipple abnormality / mass / tenderness / axillary, clavicular adenopathy
GYN/GU lesions / d/c / uterus, adnexa tenderness / CMT // circumcised / penile lesions / urethra normal location, no d/c / testes normal / + cremasteric reflex
FEET + pulses / monofilament + / nails abnormal / dry, broken skin / callus

LABS CBC / CMP / lipids / TSH / microalbumin / A1C / UA, culture / PSA / iron studies / other:

DIAGNOSTICS XR / MRI / CT / US / cardiac / other
REFERRALS   **F/U** ___ wk ___ mo

BP:	HT:
HR:	WT:
T:	BMI:
O2%:	PAIN:

NOTES . . . .

CONST	Δ appetite, energy, weight / fever / chills / sweats / fatigue
HEAD	trauma / mass / tenderness / rash / lesions
EYES	visionΔ / itch / d/c / tears / dry / cataracts / glaucoma / glasses, contacts
ENT	hearing Δ / pain / d/c / vertigo / ? infection // epistaxis / congestion // bleeding, swelling gums / pain / sore throat / voice Δ // neck pain / lumps / swelling / difficulty swallowing
CARDIAC	pain / pressure / dizzy / N / orthopnea / edema / palp / weak w exertion / hx murmurs / hx MI / HTN / HF / numb / tingle / cold extrem / slow wound healing
RESP	wheeze / SOB / cough / asthma / bronch / COPD
GI	abd pain / Δ in bowels / constipation / diarrhea / N V / hepatitis / gallstones / dysphagia / reflux / hemorrhoids / black, bloody stools
GU	burn / pain / nocturia / polyuria / hematuria / incontinence / infection / kid. stones
GENITAL	DC / sores / pain / masses / last pap ______ / sexually active Y N / dyspareunia / LMP / contraception
MSK	redness / swelling / warmth / pain / +/- ROM / arthritis / musc cramps / fracture / sprains / joint replacement / stiffness: AM PM
SKIN	rash / pruritis / jaundice / bruising / hx skin ca / mole Δ / Δ in hair, nails / lesions / slow wound healing
BREASTS	lump / pain / dc / last mammo / self exams YN
NEURO	HA / seizure / vertigo / memory Δ / gait Δ / speech / coord
PSYCH	depression / anxiety / Δ in sleep pattern / substance, ETOH abuse / suicidal ideation / homicidal ideation
ENDO	polydipsia, polyuria / heat, cold intolerance / Δ hair/nails/energy
HEM/LYMPH	anemia / bruising / hx transfusions / blood disorder / lymphadenopathy / axillary, groin tenderness
ALLX/IMMUN	season allx / food allx / med allx / immune disorder:

SOCIAL HX	# in household ______ / lives with SP/BF/GF/SO / children __ / tobacco Y/N #pk / sexual activity Y/N / etoh, other substances Y/N / occupation:
FAM HX	ca / HTN / MI / CAD / stroke / hyperlipidemia / DM2 / Alzheimer's / depression / osteoporosis / other:

GENERAL	well appearing / well nourished / a&o x 3 / normal mood / normal affect
NEURO	intact / abnormal **DTR:** 1 2 3 4 5 location:
SKIN + NAILS	turgor / rash / bruising / lesions // texture, distribution of hair // nails: abnormal color / nail deformity
HEAD	normocephalic / atraumatic / visible mass / palpable mass / depression / scarring
EYES	acuity intact / conjunctiva clear / EOM intact / PERRLA / fundi: normal discs and vessels / icterus / exudate / hemorrhage
EARS	EACs clear / TM translucent, mobile / landmarks abnormal / hearing diminished
NOSE	lesions / mucosal inflammation / septum, turbinates abnormal / sinus tenderness
MOUTH	mucous membranes dry / lesions / poor dentition / caries / gingival inflammation
PHARYNX	mucosa inflammation / tonsillar hypertrophy / tonsillar exudate
NECK	supple / ROM WNL / lesion / bruit / adenopathy / thyroid enlarged, tender / mass
CARDIAC	regular rate, rhythm / S1, S2 / murmur / gallop / click / rub / PMI displacement
RESP	clear to auscultation in all fields / wheezes (insp) (exp) / rales / crackles
ABDOMEN	BSx4 / tender / organomegaly / mass / hernia
RECTAL	abnormal tone / hemorrhoids (int/ext) / palpable mass
BACK	abnormal curvature / tenderness / CVAT / Δ ROM
EXTREMITIES	amputation / deformity / edema / varicosities / + pulses
MSK	abnormal gait / asymmetry / crepitation / defect / tenderness / mass / effusion / Δ ROM / instability / atrophy / abnormal strength, tone in head, neck, spine, ribs, pelvis, UE, LE / pathologic reflexes
PSYCH	A&O x3 / +recent/remote memory / insight / affect
BREAST	nipple abnormality / mass / tenderness / axillary, clavicular adenopathy
GYN/GU	lesions / d/c / uterus, adnexa tenderness / CMT // circumcised / penile lesions / urethra normal location, no d/c / testes normal / + cremasteric reflex
FEET	+ pulses / monofilament + / nails abnormal / dry, broken skin / callus

LABS	CBC / CMP / lipids / TSH / microalbumin / A1C / UA, culture / PSA / iron studies / other:

DIAGNOSTICS	XR / MRI / CT / US / cardiac / other
REFERRALS	**F/U** ___ wk ___ mo

Patient ID#:	**Date of visit:**
Reason for visit:	**Age: Gender:**

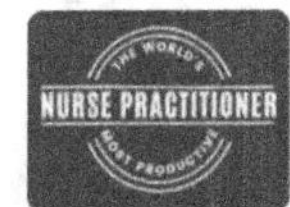

<table>
<tr><td colspan="2">

Patient ID#:
Reason for visit:

</td><td>

Date of visit:
Age: **Gender:**

</td></tr>
</table>

BP:	**HT:**
HR:	**WT:**
T:	**BMI:**
O2%:	**PAIN:**

NOTES . . . .

CONST	Δ appetite, energy, weight / fever / chills / sweats / fatigue
HEAD	trauma / mass / tenderness / rash / lesions
EYES	visionΔ / itch / d/c / tears / dry / cataracts / glaucoma / glasses, contacts
ENT	hearing Δ / pain / d/c / vertigo / ? infection // epistaxis / congestion // bleeding, swelling gums / pain / sore throat / voice Δ // neck pain / lumps / swelling / difficulty swallowing
CARDIAC	pain / pressure / dizzy / N / orthopnea / edema / palp / weak w exertion / hx murmurs / hx MI / HTN / HF / numb / tingle / cold extrem / slow wound healing
RESP	wheeze / SOB / cough / asthma / bronch / COPD
GI	abd pain / Δ in bowels / constipation / diarrhea / N V / hepatitis / gallstones / dysphagia / reflux / hemorrhoids / black, bloody stools
GU	burn / pain / nocturia / polyuria / hematuria / incontinence / infection / kid. stones
GENITAL	DC / sores / pain / masses / last pap ______ / sexually active Y N / dyspareunia / LMP ______ / contraception
MSK	redness / swelling / warmth / pain / +/- ROM / arthritis / musc cramps / fracture / sprains / joint replacement / stiffness: AM PM
SKIN	rash / pruritis / jaundice / bruising / hx skin ca / mole Δ / Δ in hair, nails / lesions / slow wound healing
BREASTS	lump / pain / dc / last mammo ______ / self exams YN
NEURO	HA / seizure / vertigo / memory Δ / gait Δ / speech / coord
PSYCH	depression / anxiety / Δ in sleep pattern / substance, ETOH abuse / suicidal ideation / homicidal ideation
ENDO	polydipsia, polyuria / heat, cold intolerance / Δ hair/nails/energy
HEM/LYMPH	anemia / bruising / hx transfusions / blood disorder / lymphadenopathy / axillary, groin tenderness
ALLX/IMMUN	season allx / food allx / med allx / immune disorder:

SOCIAL HX	# in household ______ / lives with SP/BF/GF/SO / children __ / tobacco Y/N #pk / sexual activity Y/N / etoh, other substances Y/N / occupation:
FAM HX	ca / HTN / MI / CAD / stroke / hyperlipidemia / DM2 / Alzheimer's / depression / osteoporosis / other:

GENERAL	well appearing / well nourished / a&o x 3 / normal mood / normal affect
NEURO	intact / abnormal **DTR:** 1 2 3 4 5 location:
SKIN + NAILS	turgor / rash / bruising / lesions // texture, distribution of hair // nails: abnormal color / nail deformity
HEAD	normocephalic / atraumatic / visible mass / palpable mass / depression / scarring
EYES	acuity intact / conjunctiva clear / EOM intact / PERRLA / fundi: normal discs and vessels / icterus / exudate / hemorrhage
EARS	EACs clear / TM translucent, mobile / landmarks abnormal / hearing diminished
NOSE	lesions / mucosal inflammation / septum, turbinates abnormal / sinus tenderness
MOUTH	mucous membranes dry / lesions / poor dentition / caries / gingival inflammation
PHARYNX	mucosa inflammation / tonsillar hypertrophy / tonsillar exudate
NECK	supple / ROM WNL / lesion / bruit / adenopathy / thyroid enlarged, tender / mass
CARDIAC	regular rate, rhythm / S1, S2 / murmur / gallop / click / rub / PMI displacement
RESP	clear to auscultation in all fields / wheezes (insp) (exp) / rales / crackles
ABDOMEN	BSx4 / tender / organomegaly / mass / hernia
RECTAL	abnormal tone / hemorrhoids (int/ext) / palpable mass
BACK	abnormal curvature / tenderness / CVAT / Δ ROM
EXTREMITIES	amputation / deformity / edema / varicosities / + pulses
MSK	abnormal gait / asymmetry / crepitation / defect / tenderness / mass / effusion / Δ ROM / instability / atrophy / abnormal strength, tone in head, neck, spine, ribs, pelvis, UE, LE / pathologic reflexes
PSYCH	A&O x3 / +recent/remote memory / insight / affect
BREAST	nipple abnormality / mass / tenderness / axillary, clavicular adenopathy
GYN/GU	lesions / d/c / uterus, adnexa tenderness / CMT // circumcised / penile lesions / urethra normal location, no d/c / testes normal / + cremasteric reflex
FEET	+ pulses / monofilament + / nails abnormal / dry, broken skin / callus

LABS	CBC / CMP / lipids / TSH / microalbumin / A1C / UA, culture / PSA / iron studies / other:

DIAGNOSTICS	XR / MRI / CT / US / cardiac / other
REFERRALS	

F/U ___ wk ___ mo

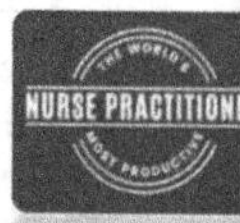

BP:	**HT:**
HR:	**WT:**
T:	**BMI:**
O2%:	**PAIN:**

<table>
<tr><td>**Patient ID#:**
Reason for visit:</td><td>**Date of visit:**
Age: **Gender:**</td></tr>
</table>

NOTES . . . .

CONST	Δ appetite, energy, weight / fever / chills / sweats / fatigue
HEAD	trauma / mass / tenderness / rash / lesions
EYES	visionΔ / itch / d/c / tears / dry / cataracts / glaucoma / glasses, contacts
ENT	hearing Δ / pain / d/c / vertigo / ? infection // epistaxis / congestion // bleeding, swelling gums / pain / sore throat / voice Δ // neck pain / lumps / swelling / difficulty swallowing
CARDIAC	pain / pressure / dizzy / N / orthopnea / edema / palp / weak w exertion / hx murmurs / hx MI / HTN / HF / numb / tingle / cold extrem / slow wound healing
RESP	wheeze / SOB / cough / asthma / bronch / COPD
GI	abd pain / Δ in bowels / constipation / diarrhea / N V / hepatitis / gallstones / dysphagia / reflux / hemorrhoids / black, bloody stools
GU	burn / pain / nocturia / polyuria / hematuria / incontinence / infection / kid. stones
GENITAL	DC / sores / pain / masses / last pap ______ / sexually active Y N / dyspareunia / LMP ______ / contraception
MSK	redness / swelling / warmth / pain / +/- ROM / arthritis / musc cramps / fracture / sprains / joint replacement / stiffness: AM PM
SKIN	rash / pruritis / jaundice / bruising / hx skin ca / mole Δ / Δ in hair, nails / lesions / slow wound healing
BREASTS	lump / pain / dc / last mammo ______ / self exams YN
NEURO	HA / seizure / vertigo / memory Δ / gait Δ / speech / coord
PSYCH	depression / anxiety / Δ in sleep pattern / substance, ETOH abuse / suicidal ideation / homicidal ideation
ENDO	polydipsia, polyuria / heat, cold intolerance / Δ hair/nails/energy
HEM/LYMPH	anemia / bruising / hx transfusions / blood disorder / lymphadenopathy / axillary, groin tenderness
ALLX/IMMUN	season allx / food allx / med allx / immune disorder:
SOCIAL HX	# in household ______ / lives with SP/BF/GF/SO / children __ / tobacco Y/N #pk / sexual activity Y/N / etoh, other substances Y/N / occupation:
FAM HX	ca / HTN / MI / CAD / stroke / hyperlipidemia / DM2 / Alzheimer's / depression / osteoporosis / other:
GENERAL	well appearing / well nourished / a&o x 3 / normal mood / normal affect
NEURO	intact / abnormal **DTR:** 1 2 3 4 5 location:
SKIN + NAILS	turgor / rash / bruising / lesions // texture, distribution of hair // nails: abnormal color / nail deformity
HEAD	normocephalic / atraumatic / visible mass / palpable mass / depression / scarring
EYES	acuity intact / conjunctiva clear / EOM intact / PERRLA / fundi: normal discs and vessels / icterus / exudate / hemorrhage
EARS	EACs clear / TM translucent, mobile / landmarks abnormal / hearing diminished
NOSE	lesions / mucosal inflammation / septum, turbinates abnormal / sinus tenderness
MOUTH	mucous membranes dry / lesions / poor dentition / caries / gingival inflammation
PHARYNX	mucosa inflammation / tonsillar hypertrophy / tonsillar exudate
NECK	supple / ROM WNL / lesion / bruit / adenopathy / thyroid enlarged, tender / mass
CARDIAC	regular rate, rhythm / S1, S2 / murmur / gallop / click / rub / PMI displacement
RESP	clear to auscultation in all fields / wheezes (insp) (exp) / rales / crackles
ABDOMEN	BSx4 / tender / organomegaly / mass / hernia
RECTAL	abnormal tone / hemorrhoids (int/ext) / palpable mass
BACK	abnormal curvature / tenderness / CVAT / Δ ROM
EXTREMITIES	amputation / deformity / edema / varicosities / + pulses
MSK	abnormal gait / asymmetry / crepitation / defect / tenderness / mass / effusion / Δ ROM / instability / atrophy / abnormal strength, tone in head, neck, spine, ribs, pelvis, UE, LE / pathologic reflexes
PSYCH	A&O x3 / +recent/remote memory / insight / affect
BREAST	nipple abnormality / mass / tenderness / axillary, clavicular adenopathy
GYN/GU	lesions / d/c / uterus, adnexa tenderness / CMT // circumcised / penile lesions / urethra normal location, no d/c / testes normal / + cremasteric reflex
FEET	+ pulses / monofilament + / nails abnormal / dry, broken skin / callus
LABS	CBC / CMP / lipids / TSH / microalbumin / A1C / UA, culture / PSA / iron studies / other:
DIAGNOSTICS	XR / MRI / CT / US / cardiac / other
REFERRALS	**F/U** ___ wk ___ mo

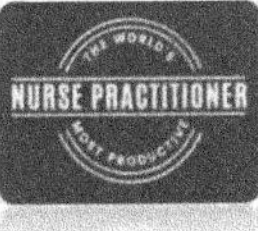

<table>
<tr><td>

Patient ID#:

Reason for visit:
</td><td>

Date of visit:

Age: **Gender:**
</td></tr>
</table>

BP: HT:
HR: WT:
T: BMI:
O2%:   PAIN:

NOTES . . . .

CONST Δ appetite, energy, weight / fever / chills / sweats / fatigue
HEAD trauma / mass / tenderness / rash / lesions
EYES visionΔ / itch / d/c / tears / dry / cataracts / glaucoma / glasses, contacts
ENT hearing Δ / pain / d/c / vertigo / ? infection // epistaxis / congestion // bleeding, swelling gums / pain / sore throat / voice Δ // neck pain / lumps / swelling / difficulty swallowing

CARDIAC pain / pressure / dizzy / N / orthopnea / edema / palp / weak w exertion / hx murmurs / hx MI / HTN / HF / numb / tingle / cold extrem / slow wound healing
RESP wheeze / SOB / cough / asthma / bronch / COPD
GI abd pain / Δ in bowels / constipation / diarrhea / N V / hepatitis / gallstones / dysphagia / reflux / hemorrhoids / black, bloody stools
GU burn / pain / nocturia / polyuria / hematuria / incontinence / infection / kid. stones
GENITAL DC / sores / pain / masses / last pap _____ / sexually active Y N / dyspareunia / LMP _____ / contraception
MSK redness / swelling / warmth / pain / +/- ROM / arthritis / musc cramps / fracture / sprains / joint replacement / stiffness: AM PM
SKIN rash / pruritis / jaundice / bruising / hx skin ca / mole Δ / Δ in hair, nails / lesions / slow wound healing
BREASTS lump / pain / dc / last mammo _____ / self exams YN
NEURO HA / seizure / vertigo / memory Δ / gait Δ / speech / coord
PSYCH depression / anxiety / Δ in sleep pattern / substance, ETOH abuse / suicidal ideation / homicidal ideation
ENDO polydipsia, polyuria / heat, cold intolerance / Δ hair/nails/energy
HEM/LYMPH anemia / bruising / hx transfusions / blood disorder / lymphadenopathy / axillary, groin tenderness
ALLX/IMMUN season allx / food allx / med allx / immune disorder:

SOCIAL HX # in household _____ / lives with SP/BF/GF/SO / children __ / tobacco Y/N #pk / sexual activity Y/N / etoh, other substances Y/N / occupation:
FAM HX ca / HTN / MI / CAD / stroke / hyperlipidemia / DM2 / Alzheimer's / depression / osteoporosis / other:

GENERAL well appearing / well nourished / a&o x 3 / normal mood / normal affect
NEURO intact / abnormal   **DTR:** 1 2 3 4 5 location:
SKIN + NAILS turgor / rash / bruising / lesions // texture, distribution of hair // nails: abnormal color / nail deformity
HEAD normocephalic / atraumatic / visible mass / palpable mass / depression / scarring
EYES acuity intact / conjunctiva clear / EOM intact / PERRLA / fundi: normal discs and vessels / icterus / exudate / hemorrhage
EARS EACs clear / TM translucent, mobile / landmarks abnormal / hearing diminished
NOSE lesions / mucosal inflammation / septum, turbinates abnormal / sinus tenderness
MOUTH mucous membranes dry / lesions / poor dentition / caries / gingival inflammation
PHARYNX mucosa inflammation / tonsillar hypertrophy / tonsillar exudate
NECK supple / ROM WNL / lesion / bruit / adenopathy / thyroid enlarged, tender / mass
CARDIAC regular rate, rhythm / S1, S2 / murmur / gallop / click / rub / PMI displacement
RESP clear to auscultation in all fields / wheezes (insp) (exp) / rales / crackles
ABDOMEN BSx4 / tender / organomegaly / mass / hernia
RECTAL abnormal tone / hemorrhoids (int/ext) / palpable mass
BACK abnormal curvature / tenderness / CVAT / Δ ROM
EXTREMITIES amputation / deformity / edema / varicosities / + pulses
MSK abnormal gait / asymmetry / crepitation / defect / tenderness / mass / effusion / Δ ROM / instability / atrophy / abnormal strength, tone in head, neck, spine, ribs, pelvis, UE, LE / pathologic reflexes
PSYCH A&O x3 / +recent/remote memory / insight / affect
BREAST nipple abnormality / mass / tenderness / axillary, clavicular adenopathy
GYN/GU lesions / d/c / uterus, adnexa tenderness / CMT // circumcised / penile lesions / urethra normal location, no d/c / testes normal / + cremasteric reflex
FEET + pulses / monofilament + / nails abnormal / dry, broken skin / callus

LABS CBC / CMP / lipids / TSH / microalbumin / A1C / UA, culture / PSA / iron studies / other:

DIAGNOSTICS XR / MRI / CT / US / cardiac / other
REFERRALS   **F/U** ___ wk ___ mo

www.ingramcontent.com/pod-product-compliance
Lightning Source LLC
Chambersburg PA
CBHW080521030726
47592CB00012B/3420